THERE ARE NO INCURABLE DISEASES

DR. RICHARD SCHULZE'S
30-Day Intensive Cleansing and Detoxification Program

NATURAL ✤ HEALING
PUBLICATIONS

Published by Natural Healing Publications
P.O. Box 3628, Santa Monica. California 90408
1-877-TEACH-ME (832-2463)

Library of Congress Catalog Card Number: 99-93974
There Are No Incurable Diseases: Dr. Richard Schulze's 30-Day
Cleansing and Detoxification Program

ISBN: 0-9671567-3-4

WARNING

A WARNING from our Lawyers:

This book is published under the First Amendment of the United States Constitution, which grants the right to discuss openly and freely all matters of public concern and to express viewpoints no matter how controversial or unaccepted they may be. However, Medical groups and Pharmaceutical companies have finally infiltrated and violated our sacred constitution. Therefore we are forced to give you the following WARNINGS:

If you are ill or have been diagnosed with any disease, please consult a medical doctor before attempting any natural healing program.

Many foods, herbs or other natural substances can occasionally have dangerous allergic reactions or side effects in some people. People have even died from allergic reactions to peanuts and strawberries.

Any one of the programs in this book could be potentially dangerous, even lethal. Especially if you are seriously ill.

Therefore, any natural method you learn about in this book may cause harm, instead of the benefit you seek. ASK YOUR DOCTOR FIRST, but remember that the vast majority of doctors have no education in natural healing methods and herbal medicine. They will probably discourage you from trying any of the programs.

DEDICATION

This book is dedicated to all my patients who had the guts, the faith and the determination to heal themselves, regardless of their medical death sentence.

I thank God that so many sick, dying souls sought me out. Together we discovered how to create healing miracles. Many literally crawled bleeding, vomiting and crying into my office. They were physically, emotionally, spiritually and financially bankrupt. They were tortured, scarred, maimed, mutilated, poisoned and burned by ignorant medical doctors until they were finally rejected and sent home to die.

But they didn't die. They pulled themselves up by what little ray of hope they had left, started on the journey to heal themselves and built a new life. Most survived and healed their so-called "incurable" diseases. Most are still alive today – healthy, disease free, happy, laughing and celebrating every day.

This book is also dedicated to those that tried and didn't make it. Those who died what I call a natural death. I love you. With many of them I was there holding their hand, talking, hugging, even singing at their last breath. Their experience helped me understand natural death. Their final words of wisdom helped me and my other patients learn how to really live.

A special thanks to Sally Wilkins, John Rizzo and Anisha Jones, my support team, who helped make this book happen.

TABLE OF CONTENTS

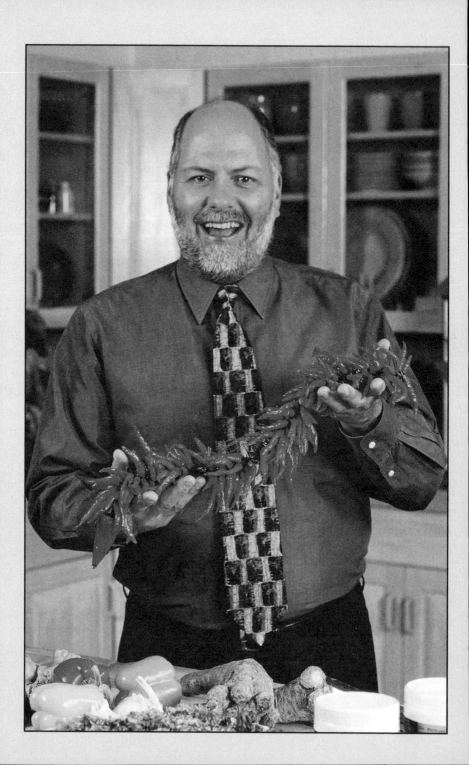

INTRODUCTION

My 30-Day Intensive Cleansing and Detoxification Program is for anyone who wants to transform their physical, emotional or spiritual health.

It doesn't matter what's wrong with you, or if anything is wrong with you at all. This program is for anyone who wants to make a dramatic change for the better in their life. In 30 days you will be a physically, emotionally and spiritually different person, a healthier person. Guaranteed!

You can custom tailor this program. You can control the level of intensity at which you want to participate. You have your foot on the gas pedal or the brake pedal. If you are just a bit run down, do the entire 30-Day Program but with the milder choices. If you are dying, turn up the intensity all the way. You have nothing to lose and everything to gain.

> **"Your body has the ability to heal itself completely of any disease."**
> **– Dr. Richard Schulze**

I was diagnosed at the age of 16 with a killer heart deformity. All my doctors agreed that I would be dead by the age of 20 unless I underwent major surgery and took prescription drugs the rest of my life. In 3 years I rebuilt my heart. I proved all the doctors wrong and so can you.

It's never too late.

I don't care how far "gone" you are. I don't care if your doctor told you there was no hope. It's never too late! You have nothing to lose and everything to gain. You just have to be READY and WILLING to change your life.

Any doubts about whether you can be totally healed and prove your doctor wrong, can hinder your progress. So if you have doubts, any doubts, you need to order a copy of my "Miracle" video **immediately!** Just call 1-877- TEACH-ME (832-2463). In this video I explain in detail my own healing miracles, why your doctors are wrong and how you can heal yourself of anything. You will also see and hear the personal testimonies of many others just like you who, against all the odds, created their own healing miracles.

Anyone with a so-called "incurable" disease needs to watch this video over and over again for positive reinforcement. You can be well. YOU CAN HEAL YOURSELF OF ANYTHING!

"There are NO 'incurable' diseases. If you are willing to take responsibility for yourself and your life, you can heal yourself of anything."
– Dr. Richard Schulze

, Arthritis, Alzheimer's Disease, Asthma, Hepatitis, AIDS, Breast Cancer, Coronary
rostate Cancer, Candida, Migraines, High Cholesterol, Endometriosis, Allergies, Poor
Disease, Memory loss, Blood Clots, Chronic Infections, Irritable Bowel Syndrome, Chr
Menopause, Herpes Simplex I II, Autoimmune Disorders, Anemia, Eczema, Epstein B
smitted Diseases, Alcoholism, Tremors, Benign Cysts and Tumors, Drug Addiction, I
Depression, Fibrocystic Breast Disease, Chronic Diarrhea, Dermatitis, Hyperthyroidis
Fibroids, Parasites, Pelvic Inflammatory Disease, Panic Attacks, Psoriasis, Lipomas,
Candida, Skin Cancer, Rheumatoid Arthritis, Congestive Heart Failure, Kidney Fail
Strokes, Panic Attacks, Hypothyroidism, Lupus, HIV, Kidney Stones, Leukemia, Ch
evere Burns, Gonorrhea, Schizophrenia, Seizures, Tuberculosis, Lead Poisoning, Poly
Disease, Multiple Sclerosis, Pyelonephritis, Pancreatic Cancer, Ulcerative Coliti
tion, Brain Cancer, Juvenile Diabetes, Mitral Valve Prolapse, Syphilis, Crohn's Dise
Addison's Disease, Cirrhosis of the Liver, Scleroderma, Ovarian Cancer, Chlamydia,
ema, Lymphoma, Lou Gehrig's Disease, Gulf War Syndrome, Glaucoma, Liver Canc
Myasthenia Gravis, Trichomonas, Nephrotic Syndrome, Rectal Cancer, Malaria, Bi
us Sclerosis, Polycystic Kidneys, Muscular Dystrophy, Lyme Disease, Sarcoidosis, Ray
Pituitary Tumors, Galactorrhea, Cystic Fibrosis, Colon Cancer, Parkinson's Disease,
ic Fatigue Syndrome, Breast Cancer, Depression, High Blood Pressure, Arthritis, Alzhe
e, Asthma, Hepatitis, Cervical Cancer, Coronary Artery Disease, Migraines, Candida
lesterol Endometriosis, Allergies, Poor Circulation, Heart Disease, Memory Loss, Blo
ic Infections, Irritable Bowel Syndrome, Chronic Sinusitis, Menopause, Herpes Simple
mmune Disorders, Anemia, Eczema, Epstein Barr, Sexually Transmitted Diseases, A
gn Cysts, Tumors, Drug Addiction, Infertility, Manic Depression, Fibrocystic Breast
ic Diarrhea, Dermatitis, Hyperthyroidism, Epilepsy, Uterine Fibroids, Parasites, Pel
Disease, Panic Attacks, Psoriasis, Lipomas, Food Allergies, Candida, Skin Cancer, R
ritis, Congestive Heart Failure, Kidney Failure, Lung Cancer, Strokes, Panic Attack
ism, Prostate Cancer, Lupus, HIV, Kidney Stones, Leukemia, Chronic Bronchitis, Se
rhea, Schizophrenia, Seizures, Tuberculosis, AIDS, Lead Poisoning, Polycystic Ovari
Multiple Sclerosis, Pyelonephritis, Pancreatic Cancer, Ulcerative Colitis, Atrial Fibrill
rain Cancer, Juvenile Diabetes, Mitral Valve Prolapse, Syphilis, Crohn's Disease, Ch
Addison's Disease, Cirrhosis of the Liver, Emphysema, Scleroderma, Ovarian Cancer,
ar Degeneration, Retinitis Pigmentosa, Lymphoma, Lou Gehrig's Disease, Gulf War
coma, Liver Cancer, Stomach Cancer, Myasthenia Gravis, Trichomonas, Nephrotic S
l Cancer, Spinal Cord Injury, Malaria, Birth Defects, Tuberous Sclerosis, Polycystic
lar Dystrophy, Lyme Disease, Sarcoidosis, Raynaud's Disease, Pituitary Tumors, Gal
Fibrosis, Colon Cancer, Parkinson's Disease, Diabetes, Chronic Fatigue Syndrome, Bre
ssion, High Blood Pressure, Arthritis, Alzheimer's Disease, Asthma, Hepatitis, Cervica
onary Artery Disease, Migraines, Candida, High Cholesterol Endometriosis, Allergie
ation, Heart Disease, Memory Loss, Blood Clots, Chronic Infections, Irritable Bowel S
ic Sinusitis, Menopause, Herpes Simplex I and II, Autoimmune Disorders, Anemia,
n Barr, Sexually Transmitted Diseases, Alcoholism, Tremors, Benign Cysts and Tum
on, Infertility, Cataracts, Macular Degeneration, Manic Depression, Fibrocystic Bre
ic Diarrhea, Dermatitis, Hyperthyroidism, Epilepsy, Uterine Fibroids, Parasites, Pelv
Disease, Panic Attacks, Psoriasis, Lipomas, Food Allergies, Candida, Skin Cancer, R
ritis, Congestive Heart Failure, Kidney Failure, Lung Cancer, Strokes, Fibromyalgia
ism, Prostate Cancer, Lupus, HIV, Kidney Stones, Leukemia, Chronic Bronchitis, Se
hea, Schizophrenia, Seizures, Tuberculosis, AIDS, Lead Poisoning, Polycystic Ovari

CHAPTER 1

WHAT THIS PROGRAM WILL DO FOR YOU

PHYSICALLY

Modern life exposes us to literally thousands of different poisons and toxins every day. The average grocery cart alone has over 100 toxic chemicals in it. It is no secret that the quality of our food, water and air have degenerated, especially in the last 25 years.

Additionally, during the normal metabolic functions of our body, we create many different types of waste like urine, feces, mucous, acids, bile, pus, etc... Modern living with its lack of exercise and above average levels of stress, inhibits our body's natural ability to remove waste. **The build up of these toxins and waste in our body is killing us and directly causes Cancer, Heart Disease, Neuromuscular Disease, Digestive Disease, Diabetes, Arthritis, and a thousand other diseases.**

This program is a strong, detoxifying flush. It will draw, vacuum out and facilitate the removal of old accumulated poisons and toxic chemicals. It will eliminate and purge them from all the places they like to hide in your body like your fat, muscles, intestines, liver, gall bladder, kidneys, bloodstream, lymphatic system, tissues and cells.

This program will also stimulate and boost your immune system. It will give your body the nutrition to build itself back up and heal disease.

Many quick cleanses and 24 hour detoxes claim magical results but the only potency is in their advertising. After 30 or 40 years of typical American degenerative living, do you really think you can reverse all the damage and get rid of all the built up muck in a day or two? If so then I have some oceanfront property in Arizona I would like to sell you.

This program has proven itself in my clinic spanning 2 decades to beneficially affect every part, every organ, every system, every joint, every cell in your body. It gets the accumulated gunk (that's a medical term) out and the nutrition in.

After doing this program, people often remark that they have incredible energy and that they look and feel better than they have in 30 years. That's not a bad trade off – a year for each day on the program.

After 30 days, most of my patients' complaints, problems and diseases were gone.

EMOTIONALLY

Your brain is an organ just like any other organ in your body. It can only work well when it is supplied with sufficient blood and that blood must be rich in nutrients. Your brain also creates waste as it works – thinking, problem solving, meditating or stimulating millions of nerves cells or manufacturing numerous metabolic chemicals that tell your body to do everything from balancing your hormones to recovering from jet lag.

Often, while viewing an autopsy that opens the skull and dissects the brain, or when reading a post mortem pathology report, some part of the the brain tissue is usually anemic and physically covered with yellow mucous and waste. This proves the lack of blood and the retention of waste. When viewing the brain of someone with a brain disease, the brain usually looks even worse.

Medical doctors and scientists would like to make this more complicated. It isn't. From slight memory loss to Alzheimer's disease, from bad days to chronic depression, even insanity, **ALL** brain and emotional dysfunction has its roots in bad circulation, nutritional depletion and waste build up.

SPIRITUALLY

Moses, Jesus, Buddha, Mohammed, Krishna and other prophets, saints, and spiritual leaders and even entire organized religions – from the Mormons to the Methodists – preach fasting, nutrition, cleansing and detoxification for clarity. Since ancient times, fasting, cleansing with herbs and even giving enemas with hollowed out gourds has been practiced to increase spiritual ability and closeness to God.

Whatever your spiritual beliefs or religion – from Adventists to Zen – my 30-Day Cleansing and Detoxification Program will increase your ability to hear and understand the Word of God, to receive divine messages and let God work through you. Hallelujah!

re, Arthritis, Alzheimer's Disease, Asthma, Hepatitis, AIDS, Breast Cancer, Coronar
rostate Cancer, Candida, Migraines, High Cholesterol, Endometriosis, Allergies, Poor
Disease, Memory loss, Blood Clots, Chronic Infections, Irritable Bowel Syndrome, Chr
Menopause, Herpes Simplex I II, Autoimmune Disorders, Anemia, Eczema, Epstein B
smitted Diseases, Alcoholism, Tremors, Benign Cysts and Tumors, Drug Addiction, I
Depression, Fibrocystic Breast Disease, Chronic Diarrhea, Dermatitis, Hyperthyroidi
Fibroids, Parasites, Pelvic Inflammatory Disease, Panic Attacks, Psoriasis, Lipomas,
Candida, Skin Cancer, Rheumatoid Arthritis, Congestive Heart Failure, Kidney Fai
Strokes, Panic Attacks, Hypothyroidism, Lupus, HIV, Kidney Stones, Leukemia, Ch
evere Burns, Gonorrhea, Schizophrenia, Seizures, Tuberculosis, Lead Poisoning, Poly
Disease, Multiple Sclerosis, Pyelonephritis, Pancreatic Cancer, Ulcerative Colitis
ation, Brain Cancer, Juvenile Diabetes, Mitral Valve Prolapse, Syphilis, Crohn's Dise
Addison's Disease, Cirrhosis of the Liver, Scleroderma, Ovarian Cancer, Chlamydia
sema, Lymphoma, Lou Gehrig's Disease, Gulf War Syndrome, Glaucoma, Liver Canc
Myasthenia Gravis, Trichomonas, Nephrotic Syndrome, Rectal Cancer, Malaria, B
us Sclerosis, Polycystic Kidneys, Muscular Dystrophy, Lyme Disease, Sarcoidosis, Ray
Pituitary Tumors, Galactorrhea, Cystic Fibrosis, Colon Cancer, Parkinson's Disease,
ic Fatigue Syndrome, Breast Cancer, Depression, High Blood Pressure, Arthritis, Alzhe
e, Asthma, Hepatitis, Cervical Cancer, Coronary Artery Disease, Migraines, Candid
lesterol Endometriosis, Allergies, Poor Circulation, Heart Disease, Memory Loss, Blo
ic Infections, Irritable Bowel Syndrome, Chronic Sinusitis, Menopause, Herpes Simple
mmune Disorders, Anemia, Eczema, Epstein Barr, Sexually Transmitted Diseases, A
ign Cysts, Tumors, Drug Addiction, Infertility, Manic Depression, Fibrocystic Breast
ic Diarrhea, Dermatitis, Hyperthyroidism, Epilepsy, Uterine Fibroids, Parasites, Pel
Disease, Panic Attacks, Psoriasis, Lipomas, Food Allergies, Candida, Skin Cancer, R
ritis, Congestive Heart Failure, Kidney Failure, Lung Cancer, Strokes, Panic Attack
ism, Prostate Cancer, Lupus, HIV, Kidney Stones, Leukemia, Chronic Bronchitis, Se
rhea, Schizophrenia, Seizures, Tuberculosis, AIDS, Lead Poisoning, Polycystic Ovari
ultiple Sclerosis, Pyelonephritis, Pancreatic Cancer, Ulcerative Colitis, Atrial Fibrill
rain Cancer, Juvenile Diabetes, Mitral Valve Prolapse, Syphilis, Crohn's Disease, Ch
Addison's Disease, Cirrhosis of the Liver, Emphysema, Scleroderma, Ovarian Cancer,
ar Degeneration, Retinitis Pigmentosa, Lymphoma, Lou Gehrig's Disease, Gulf War
coma, Liver Cancer, Stomach Cancer, Myasthenia Gravis, Trichomonas, Nephrotic S
l Cancer, Spinal Cord Injury, Malaria, Birth Defects, Tuberous Sclerosis, Polycystic
lar Dystrophy, Lyme Disease, Sarcoidosis, Raynaud's Disease, Pituitary Tumors, Gal
ibrosis, Colon Cancer, Parkinson's Disease, Diabetes, Chronic Fatigue Syndrome, Bre
ssion, High Blood Pressure, Arthritis, Alzheimer's Disease, Asthma, Hepatitis, Cervica
onary Artery Disease, Migraines, Candida, High Cholesterol Endometriosis, Allergie
ation, Heart Disease, Memory Loss, Blood Clots, Chronic Infections, Irritable Bowel S
ic Sinusitis, Menopause, Herpes Simplex I and II, Autoimmune Disorders, Anemia,
n Barr, Sexually Transmitted Diseases, Alcoholism, Tremors, Benign Cysts and Tumo
on, Infertility, Cataracts, Macular Degeneration, Manic Depression, Fibrocystic Brea
c Diarrhea, Dermatitis, Hyperthyroidism, Epilepsy, Uterine Fibroids, Parasites, Pelv
Disease, Panic Attacks, Psoriasis, Lipomas, Food Allergies, Candida, Skin Cancer, R
ritis, Congestive Heart Failure, Kidney Failure, Lung Cancer, Strokes, Fibromyalgia
ism, Prostate Cancer, Lupus, HIV, Kidney Stones, Leukemia, Chronic Bronchitis, Se
hea, Schizophrenia, Seizures, Tuberculosis, AIDS, Lead Poisoning, Polycystic Ovarie
Sclerosis, Pyelonephritis, Pancreatic Cancer, Ulcerative Colitis, Atrial Fibrill

CHAPTER 2

THERE ARE NO INCURABLE DISEASES

> "Your body has a blueprint, a schematic of what perfect health is and is constantly trying to achieve this perfect health for you."
> — Dr. Richard Schulze

YOU ARE NOT THE EXCEPTION TO THE RULE

I know you think your disease is unique or different. IT ISN'T. I know you think I am talking about most diseases or only killer diseases *but certainly not yours.* I AM TALKING ABOUT YOUR DISEASE.

I am talking about EVERY disease including Arthritis, Stomach Ulcers, Digestive Complaints, Constipation, Diabetes, Alzheimer's, High Blood Pressure, ALL Cancers, Parkinson's Disease, Heart Disease, Chronic Fatigue, Lupus, Depression, Neurologic Diseases, Muscular Diseases, Skin Diseases, Emotional Diseases and even diseases that no one has discovered or named yet.

Even if your great, highly-educated medical doctor says that your disease is "incurable," that there is NO CURE and that NOTHING CAN BE DONE, or that there is no cure EXCEPT their treatment, THEY ARE WRONG. Maybe they even say you will be dead in a few months, or weeks. BULL!

I had patients that were told by their doctors, the greatest medical specialists in the country, the *"top guns,"* that they would be dead in a few weeks or a month at best. Many who came to me were literally crawling up the stairs suffering from severe heart damage with 90% artery blockage, from last stage A.I.D.S. with 1 or 2 T-cells left, from all types of Cancer and Leukemia with anemia so bad they were bleeding through the skin, or from Arthritis so painful it hurt them to breathe. Others were suffocating with lung disease, convulsing with spasms or paralyzed with neuromuscular diseases.

THESE PATIENTS ARE STILL ALIVE TODAY, 15 YEARS LATER. No, they were not misdiagnosed. It was not a spontaneous remission. It was not a fluke that they lived, thrived and celebrated long, healthy, vital, happy lives. THEY HEALED THEMSELVES!

Get my point?

I don't give a damn what name your doctors put on your disease, I don't care how "incurable" or potentially deadly they say it is and I could care less how highly educated your doctors are, how many degrees they have or how many books they've written. They have long forgotten their first day in medical school where they learned that the body's first and foremost job is to survive and repair itself. As long as you are still breathing, I am going to show you how to make your doctors eat their words. I am going to teach you how to increase your body's ability to survive and repair itself beyond your doctors' wildest imagination, beyond anything they learned in medical school, beyond what any of them believe the human body is capable of. I am going to teach you how to create a healing miracle.

My patients that really wanted to be well and had the guts, faith and determination to follow the programs, healed themselves.

DO IT NOW

Take responsibility for yourself. Take a look in the mirror. This is the person who is responsible for your current health. YOU are the ONLY

ONE who can help you. You created this problem and you can heal yourself. So take a deep breath. Get a grip. Stop feeling sorry for yourself and get to work creating your new life.

A great scholar once said that "sympathy" lies between "shit" and "syphilis" in the dictionary. Well, wherever it lies, I never saw it help even one of my patients get better. No one ever got better by feeling sorry for themselves.

So what are you waiting for? Get up off your sick butt, put the sleeping pills or gun away and give me 110%. Take responsibility for your life. Take your life back into your own hands. You will be amazed at the miracle healing that will happen to you. **YOU CAN DO IT!!!!**

Maybe you have tried every supplement or drug.

I know your kitchen cupboards are overflowing with everything from vitamins, minerals, herbs and enzymes to amino acids, melatonin, shark cartilage, colloidal silver, glucosamine sulfate, and every other natural fad. I know your medicine cabinet is filled with prescription drugs, over the counter drugs and even some your friends gave you. I know your nightstand next to your bed is filled with this same stuff. Nothing has worked and you're getting sicker. **This program WILL work for you.**

Maybe you have tried the best medical doctors.

The medical doctors tried to kill your disease without your help. This almost never works and when it does, it is only a temporary, quick fix. I am not going to kill or even cure your disease. I am going to get you so healthy, your disease is going to run, leap and jump out of your body. I will not lie to you like your medical doctors and pretend to know the intricate functions of your body. Only God knows that. However, I do know that if I get you to create an extremely healthy lifestyle, one beyond your wildest imagination, your body will heal itself.

Maybe you have even tried every natural doctor.

They are all a big bunch of wimps, especially when it comes to turning up the intensity.

The reason my patients were able to heal their so-called "incurable" diseases, the reason my patients created healing miracles is because **I didn't stop kicking their asses until they were well.**

Natural and alternative doctors fool around balancing your aura and spritzing you with essential oils – what I call "finishing treatments." Even if they get tough, they still use wimpy programs with impotent, pathetic dosages. At least a medical doctor knows how to treat killer diseases with intensity. They will cut the top of your head off and carve a tumor out, cut your testicles off or yank out your ovaries. Get it? If you are going to heal yourself of a killer disease with natural healing instead of modern medicine, you have to pull out all the stops. Turn the intensity up to 110%. Put the pedal to the metal and don't look back.

I never killed any of my patients.

No, I never killed a one, but I pushed the limits and took all my natural healing methods to the MAX. I may have turned some of my patients inside out with wheatgrass juice or the Cold Sheet Treatment but I never killed or even hurt one of them. I never put too much ice in the ice bath, or pushed them too hard in their emotional healing. I never gave them too much cayenne pepper, purged them too much, cleansed them too much, or had one die from a juice overdose. I tried, but they didn't break. I dared some of them to go ahead and die on me, but they didn't. THEY LIVED, THRIVED AND CELEBRATED LONG, HEALTHY, VITAL, HAPPY LIVES. **THEY HEALED THEMSELVES!**

> **"Your body has the ability to completely heal itself. It just needs your assistance."**
>
> **– Dr. Richard Schulze**

No one is dying from over zealous natural doctors, over intense programs or overdoses of herbs. They are dying from not enough!

When I visit my students' clinics in America, Europe, anywhere in the world, they often line up their worst cases for me in the hallway. These were the patients they hadn't been able to cure – patients that were not responding to treatment.

99% of the time my student doctors were doing all the right things, just not enough of them and not often enough. I always tell them, "TURN UP THE DARN INTENSITY."

The main problem is that most natural doctors are afraid of hurting someone. They don't want to break the patient – to push them too far. If a patient has a terminal, "incurable" or killer disease, YOU HAVE TO TURN UP THE INTENSITY. GO AHEAD. TRY TO KILL THEM WITH CARROT JUICE, ENEMAS, HERBAL PURGES AND POSITIVE THINKING. YOU CAN'T.

I would scream at these doctors, "What are you afraid of? Killing them? They are already dying. You have nothing to lose."

Often I would take what the doctor had the patient doing in one day and make them do it in an hour, and then repeat it 8 or 10 more times that day. Push it to the MAX!

People are much tougher than you think.

When I would look into the lives of these supposedly frail patients, the way they lived and took care of themselves before they got sick was very intense. These people were drinking pints of harmful beverages, smoking cigarettes and on a steady diet of animal foods and bad attitudes. They never questioned all the ways they were trying to kill themselves. They never questioned when they opened their seventh beer why beer comes in six-packs and maybe seven is an overdose. They just chugged it down.

They never questioned that maybe one bag of greasy potato chips or junk snacks was a dosage when they ripped open the next bag, munched it down and changed the TV channel. They didn't call the manufacturer to see if maybe they were over doing it. They just partied hearty.

Cigarettes, Booze, Coffee, Sugar, Chocolate, Fast Food, Recreational Drugs, Prescription Drugs, Artificial Everything, Household Toxins, Environmental Pollutants, Bad Relationships and Filling Our Minds With Garbage – WE NEVER QUESTIONED IT. WE NEVER SLOWED DOWN. WE NEVER WORRIED ABOUT OVERDOSE.

BUT NOW, in healing ourselves, we are concerned about taking an over dose of herbs. We are worried that one too many cups of ginger root tea in the Cold Sheet Treatment will be too rough. GIVE ME A BREAK!

If people used half as much determination, energy and intensity healing themselves as they used partying, tearing themselves down and trying to kill themselves, they could have healing miracles, almost immediately.

Maybe you have tried every health program.
Maybe you have tried hundreds of different health programs, routines and formulae. Have you ever done them all at once? I am going to ask you to fill your days and nights with healing routines. It will be your full time job for the next 30-days. If you are really ill, quit your job or take a leave of absence. You have to give this program 110%. You will have to put yourself before anything else.

Get a healing partner.
Your chances of success are 1000 times better if you have a friend to assist you. Why do an enema all by yourself? You will mess up the whole bathroom and it will take all night long. Invite a friend.

If you are em-bare-assed, (no pun intended), get over it. This will be part of your healing. The fun is just beginning.

Rarely should this helper be your spouse. They are either too close to you to kick your ass when you need it or maybe you are sick because they have been kicking your ass too much all your life. Again your spouse is almost always a bad choice and I advise against it.

Find a friend, relative or, even better, someone you met at the health food store who is also interested in health and natural healing. Most importantly this person has to be strong, have a firm hand, be able to lift your spirits when they are down, laugh if you poop your pants, even cry with you and then get up and be excited and ready to do it all over again.

> "Getting well is easy, it is getting sick that takes years of constant, dedicated hard work."
>
> – Dr. Richard Schulze

ostate Cancer, Candida, Migraines, High Cholesterol, Endometriosis, Allergies, Poor
Disease, Memory loss, Blood Clots, Chronic Infections, Irritable Bowel Syndrome, Ch
Menopause, Herpes Simplex I II, Autoimmune Disorders, Anemia, Eczema, Epstein B
smitted Diseases, Alcoholism, Tremors, Benign Cysts and Tumors, Drug Addiction,
Depression, Fibrocystic Breast Disease, Chronic Diarrhea, Dermatitis, Hyperthyroidi
Fibroids, Parasites, Pelvic Inflammatory Disease, Panic Attacks, Psoriasis, Lipomas,
Candida, Skin Cancer, Rheumatoid Arthritis, Congestive Heart Failure, Kidney Fail
Strokes, Panic Attacks, Hypothyroidism, Lupus, HIV, Kidney Stones, Leukemia, Ch
vere Burns, Gonorrhea, Schizophrenia, Seizures, Tuberculosis, Lead Poisoning, Poly
Disease, Multiple Sclerosis, Pyelonephritis, Pancreatic Cancer, Ulcerative Colitis
tion, Brain Cancer, Juvenile Diabetes, Mitral Valve Prolapse, Syphilis, Crohn's Dise
Addison's Disease, Cirrhosis of the Liver, Scleroderma, Ovarian Cancer, Chlamydia,
ma, Lymphoma, Lou Gehrig's Disease, Gulf War Syndrome, Glaucoma, Liver Canc
Myasthenia Gravis, Trichomonas, Nephrotic Syndrome, Rectal Cancer, Malaria, B
us Sclerosis, Polycystic Kidneys, Muscular Dystrophy, Lyme Disease, Sarcoidosis, Ray
Pituitary Tumors, Galactorrhea, Cystic Fibrosis, Colon Cancer, Parkinson's Disease,
c Fatigue Syndrome, Breast Cancer, Depression, High Blood Pressure, Arthritis, Alzhe
, Asthma, Hepatitis, Cervical Cancer, Coronary Artery Disease, Migraines, Candid
esterol Endometriosis, Allergies, Poor Circulation, Heart Disease, Memory Loss, Blo
c Infections, Irritable Bowel Syndrome, Chronic Sinusitis, Menopause, Herpes Simple
mmune Disorders, Anemia, Eczema, Epstein Barr, Sexually Transmitted Diseases, A
n Cysts, Tumors, Drug Addiction, Infertility, Manic Depression, Fibrocystic Breast
c Diarrhea, Dermatitis, Hyperthyroidism, Epilepsy, Uterine Fibroids, Parasites, Pel
Disease, Panic Attacks, Psoriasis, Lipomas, Food Allergies, Candida, Skin Cancer,
itis, Congestive Heart Failure, Kidney Failure, Lung Cancer, Strokes, Panic Attacks
sm, Prostate Cancer, Lupus, HIV, Kidney Stones, Leukemia, Chronic Bronchitis, Se
hea, Schizophrenia, Seizures, Tuberculosis, AIDS, Lead Poisoning, Polycystic Ovaria
ultiple Sclerosis, Pyelonephritis, Pancreatic Cancer, Ulcerative Colitis, Atrial Fibrilla
rain Cancer, Juvenile Diabetes, Mitral Valve Prolapse, Syphilis, Crohn's Disease, Ch
ddison's Disease, Cirrhosis of the Liver, Emphysema, Scleroderma, Ovarian Cancer,
r Degeneration, Retinitis Pigmentosa, Lymphoma, Lou Gehrig's Disease, Gulf War
oma, Liver Cancer, Stomach Cancer, Myasthenia Gravis, Trichomonas, Nephrotic Sy
Cancer, Spinal Cord Injury, Malaria, Birth Defects, Tuberous Sclerosis, Polycystic
ar Dystrophy, Lyme Disease, Sarcoidosis, Raynaud's Disease, Pituitary Tumors, Gal
ibrosis, Colon Cancer, Parkinson's Disease, Diabetes, Chronic Fatigue Syndrome, Bre
sion, High Blood Pressure, Arthritis, Alzheimer's Disease, Asthma, Hepatitis, Cervica
nary Artery Disease, Migraines, Candida, High Cholesterol Endometriosis, Allergie
tion, Heart Disease, Memory Loss, Blood Clots, Chronic Infections, Irritable Bowel S
ic Sinusitis, Menopause, Herpes Simplex I and II, Autoimmune Disorders, Anemia,
Barr, Sexually Transmitted Diseases, Alcoholism, Tremors, Benign Cysts and Tumo
n, Infertility, Cataracts, Macular Degeneration, Manic Depression, Fibrocystic Brea
Diarrhea, Dermatitis, Hyperthyroidism, Epilepsy, Uterine Fibroids, Parasites, Pelv
Disease, Panic Attacks, Psoriasis, Lipomas, Food Allergies, Candida, Skin Cancer,
itis, Congestive Heart Failure, Kidney Failure, Lung Cancer, Strokes, Fibromyalgia,
m, Prostate Cancer, Lupus, HIV, Kidney Stones, Leukemia, Chronic Bronchitis, Sei
ea, Schizophrenia, Seizures, Tuberculosis, AIDS, Lead Poisoning, Polycystic Ovaria

CHAPTER 3

THE 30-DAY JUICE/FOOD PROGRAM

For 30 days you will be consuming only pure water, herbal teas, fresh fruit and vegetable juices, and raw foods including fruits, vegetables, seeds, sprouts, nuts, legumes and grains.

To increase the effectiveness of the program, I suggest you consume only liquids for 2-3 consecutive days each week.

If you are seriously ill, you must do a fresh juice flush for the entire month. No solid food!

GET A JUICER TODAY

Owning a juicer is mandatory. It is not an option! If you don't have one, buy one today. It will save your life. I don't care what kind or what make it is. Sure, some juicers are better than others but let's not miss the point. GET A JUICER AND START USING IT TODAY. Without a juicer, forget doing this program.

Drink at least one gallon of liquid a day. That's eight 16-ounce servings. Use only distilled or purified water, Detoxification Herb Tea, herbal teas (non-caffeine) and organic fruit and vegetable juices. You can dilute your juice with 50% distilled or purified water if this feels right to you. I rarely saw any patients have any significant problems with the natural sugars present in juices – even Diabetics. If someone did have a problem, diluting the juice with 50% pure water eliminated it.

Don't think of this as a juice *fast,* but instead a JUICE FLUSH. You will literally be pouring gallons of nutritional, vital, healing, cleansing, strengthening and potent juices into your body, into your bloodstream and into every cell of your body, replacing old fluids. This is the greatest oil change in the world.

Organic produce is obviously the best way to go because most pesticides and insecticides are poisonous and hurt your immune system and your nervous system. If you can't get organic, don't let that stop you. Just soak and wash the produce if you feel it might be contaminated. Inferior produce making less potent juice is still better than not juicing. Don't look for reasons to not do the program. Just do the best you can. Get the freshest, most vital, cleanest, most nutritious produce you can find. I even had patients heal themselves of "incurable" diseases using leftover scraps from the Farmer's Market.

These days, most communities have local farmers' markets. These are usually the best place to find fresh, organic produce.

> **"Getting well is just a matter of stopping what you did that made you sick and starting new programs that create health."**
> **– Dr. Richard Schulze**

TIPS TO HELP YOU SUCCEED ON YOUR JUICE FLUSH:

Your Body Temperature

When you do a juice flush, you will naturally be consuming less calories, or heat units. Occasionally during your flush, you will feel a bit cooler than normal. Maybe you'll even get an occasional shiver or chill depending on the time of year you do your flush. This is no problem. I would always tell my patients to keep a sweatshirt in the back of their car or with them all the time so if they felt a bit cooler they could throw it on. Usually during a flush, if you go out or to work, you want to have a backpack with you anyway, to keep extra juice or water with you. Just keep a sweater, light jacket, whatever, in your backpack.

Your Energy Level

When you are consuming less food, or no food, you may experience occasional energy lulls. You may suddenly feel like, "I have no energy in my body. I can't get up." Relax. Don't panic. This feeling will only last a few minutes and then you will have more energy than you know what to do with. Short, temporary, energy dips are common when flushing, especially during a 30-Day juice flush without any solid food. But intense energy BLASTS are even more common.

On the 28th day of one of my personal 30-Day juice flushes, I was supposed to drive an hour to a gym and kick-box which takes a lot of energy, much more than regular boxing. I didn't feel up to it. I felt out of energy but I dragged myself there anyway. After pushing myself through 30 minutes of warm up exercises, it was like I was suddenly on rocket fuel instead of only juice. I kick-boxed 17 three-minute rounds. I was better than ever, a personal best. When it was all over one of the top instructors came over to me and said, "I don't know what you're on, but you were moving so fast we could hardly see you! You were like a blur!" So much for a lack of energy when juice flushing.

Hunger Panic

Occasionally during a juice flush you will have an intense and immediate craving for food. They can seem very intense momentarily and you want to run to the kitchen and EAT everything in sight. Well DON'T.

These are just temporary metabolic shifts in your body. Don't attach to them and they will be gone in minutes, if not seconds.

You should never feel hungry on a juice flush. If you do, you need to drink more liquid. If you still feel hungry, wait a few minutes, drink more and keep drinking more until you are full.

MORNING NUTRITIONAL DRINK

Nature has blessed us with certain foods and herbs that are extremely potent, concentrated and complete. I call them SUPERFOODS. I designed this organic, concentrated, natural vitamin and mineral mixture for my sickest patients. Often, when you are really ill, your digestive system is also in poor working order. You can hardly digest and assimilate anything. My SuperFood formula is packed with single celled plants and the beauty is they almost digest themselves. In minutes you have a blast of vitamins and minerals in your blood stream, building and healing your body. My SuperFood created more miracles in my clinic than any of my other herbal formulae. To this day, I get letters and calls every week from customers raving about how this simple drink gives them more energy and vitality than they have had in years. It is life changing.

Getting that extra boost from these SUPERFOODS is the missing link that many have been searching for and their bodies have been begging for. Consume 2 nutritional drinks daily, one in the morning and one in the early afternoon. Some people say it keeps them awake at night if they drink it too late in the day. It contains no caffeine or stimulants of any kind. It is just that that your brain loves this potent nutritional blast and you end up contemplating world peace instead of sleeping.

Mix in a blender:
- 8 ounces of fresh squeezed fruit or vegetable juice
- 8 ounces of distilled or purified water
- If you are eating solid food, include 1/2-1 cup of fresh seasonal fruit or vegetables. (Fruits and vegetables that are put in a blender rather than a juicer still have all the fiber in them and we consider this more like a solid food.)
- 2 heaping tablespoons of Dr. Schulze's SuperFood. Remember, juices are a natural healing blood transfusion. I have seen miracles in a matter of hours using juices.

One of the most powerful healing, blood building and cleansing juice combinations is:
- 12 ounces of carrot juice
- 2 ounces of beet root juice
- 1 ounce of beet green juice
- 1 ounce of wheatgrass juice
- 2 heaping tablespoons of **Dr. Schulze's SuperFood**

How to get **Dr. Schulze's SuperFood?** See the supplier section in the back of this book.

IF YOU HAVE DECIDED TO EAT...

EVERYTHING MUST BE VEGAN AND RAW

If you are not seriously ill and have decided to eat solid food during your 30-Day Program, then all food consumed must be 100% Vegan and 100% raw, (not cooked or heated in any way.) This includes all fresh fruits, vegetables, seeds, sprouts, nuts, legumes and grains. Everything must be eaten raw, or soaked and sprouted. Eat fresh organic produce that is grown locally and in season. Drink only distilled or purified water, herbal teas (non-caffeinated) and fruit and vegetable juices.

Even if you decide to eat raw foods you still must drink as much fresh juice as possible – at least 64 ounces a day. Absolutely NO animal flesh, eggs, milk, or milk products (cheese, yogurt or butter.) No cooked foods, (bread, pasta, baked potatoes, tofu, etc.....) NO alcohol, coffee, black tea or sugar.

WHAT TO EAT

1. Raw vegetables and vegetable juices: A juicer and blender are the best investments for your future health and vitality. Don't forget good vegetables like potatoes, turnips, carrots, beets, dark greens, as well as the cruciferous vegetables like cabbage, cauliflower, broccoli, brussels sprouts and kale. How about raw corn, on or off the cob, peas, green beans and squashes of all types. Don't be afraid to use onions (all types; green, red and white), hot peppers and TONS of garlic. Let's make some sprouts - mung, alfalfa, red clover, sunflower, lentil, wheat and garbanzo. Soak your beans (all types) and try blending them with some olive oil, garlic and spices to make homemade raw hummus. GREENS: Forget iceberg lettuce; how about some red and green cabbage, spinach, romaine, chard, collards, mustard, turnip and dandelion.

2. Fresh fruits and fruit juices: Melons are very high in vitamins and minerals, (watermelon, honeydew, cantaloupes, crenshaw, etc...) Papaya, mangoes, pineapple, bananas, cherries, plums, prunes, raisins, grapes, pears, figs, dates, oranges, limes, lemons, grapefruit (red, pink and white), tangerines, berries (strawberries, blackberries, raspberries, blueberries), avocado, apricots, peaches, nectarines, and last but not least, all the beautiful types of apples.

3. Nuts and seeds: (Raw and unsalted only.) Some good ones are brazil nuts, almonds, pecans, walnuts, filberts and pepitas. Make your own raw nut butter in a blender, adding some maple syrup. Some good seeds are sunflower, sesame, pumpkin and flax.

4. Beans and grains: Soak and sprout, then eat as sprouts. You can make grain and seed dehydrated breads. No cooking or baking.

WHAT NOT TO EAT
Do not eat any animal's flesh, limbs, internal organs, fetuses or milk. In other words, don't eat any cows, lambs, pigs, birds, ducks, chickens, turkeys, fish, rabbits, frogs, turtles, snails, etc... No animal scavengers, (clams, lobster, shrimp, oysters, etc.....)

Do not eat any heated grains or grain products, (brown rice, breads, crackers, muffins, pitas, tofu, commercial cereals, commercially prepared fake meat soy products or wheat substitutes.)

Don't consume any coffee, caffeine tea, alcohol, tobacco, sugar, salt, drugs, artificial sweeteners, colors, flavors, preservatives, insecticides or chemicals of any kind. Don't eat any processed foods, canned foods or commercially frozen food. All unrefrigerated bottled juices are pasteurized (cooked). I consider them colored mineral water – O.K. but not vital.

If in doubt, DON'T EAT IT. Have a glass of juice... Watch out when eating in restaurants, even so-called "Health Food" ones. Most of the waiters and waitresses don't know exactly what is in the food, so ask a chef or cook if you can. Never assume anything. A good restaurant won't object to your inquiries.

Garlic

Consume at least 3 cloves of fresh raw garlic every day.

If you do only one program and use only one herb, it should be garlic. Over the years in the clinic, I have seen garlic heal many, hurt no one, and create miracles.

Garlic is one of the most potent and reliable herbal healers known. It is a powerful broad spectrum antibiotic. Besides being anti-bacterial, it is also anti-viral, anti-fungal, anti-parasitic and has proven itself to rid the body internally and externally of any antigens or pathogens.

Garlic has been proven in hospitals and laboratories worldwide to destroy cancer and break up tumors, thin the blood and normalize blood pressure and cholesterol levels.

Hundreds of my female patients use vaginal garlic implants to do everything from heal infections to eliminate cancer.

Externally, garlic is an herbal surgeon. Its 75 various sulphur compounds will destroy infections, and if used full strength, will burn off anything in its way.

Nutritionally, garlic is a great strength builder and has been revered throughout history in many cultures as a way to increase health and energy.

Garlic can be eaten raw, swallowed whole, chopped up and mixed with food and put through your juicer. Just get it in. The best garlic is the hottest and, of course, organic. If none is available, which is rare, use your hottest onions, which is garlic's next of kin.

We had a lady call and say, "I don't like garlic. It makes me smell bad." Anisha, my partner, overheard the conversation and yelled, "Then don't get well!" If you want to undertake natural healing, don't be whining about the garlic odor on your breath with your social friends. I mean, we're talking about saving someone's life here!

Potassium Broth Recipe

Potassium Broth is a great-tasting addition to your cleansing program. It will flush your system of toxins, poisons and unwanted salts and acids while giving you a concentrated amount of vitamins and minerals. Drink as much as you can stand. Make a large pot once or twice a week. USE ORGANIC PRODUCE ONLY.

Fill a large pot with:
- 25% potato peelings,
- 25% carrot peelings and whole chopped beets
- 25% chopped onions
- 25% celery and dark greens
- 50 cloves of garlic, minimum,
- Hot peppers to taste
- Enough distilled water to cover vegetables

Simmer on very low temperature for 2 hours or more. Strain, or just dip your mug in, and drink only the broth. Put the vegetables in your compost. Make enough for 2 days, refrigerating the leftover broth. It is important to use organic vegetables. We do not want to consume any toxic insecticides, pesticides or inorganic chemical fertilizers while we are on a cleansing and detoxification program.

GOOD SUPPLEMENTS / ADDITIONS

- Organic, extra virgin, cold pressed, unfiltered olive oil
- Organic, raw, unfiltered apple cider vinegar
- Cayenne pepper and garlic

BAD SUPPLEMENTS

- Salt of any kind. Commercial soy sauce (tamari) and miso. They are loaded with salt. Also, watch out for kelp. Kelp in its natural state is not extremely salty. If yours is, then it has sea salt in it, which is just as unassimilable as all salt.
- Vitamin, mineral and nutritional supplements taken from animal or inorganic sources, (e.g...fish liver oils, glandular formulas, some digestive enzymes, mineral tablets, etc...)
- Don't eat anything isolated or not in its wholesome organic state.

rostate Cancer, Candida, Migraines, High Cholesterol, Endometriosis, Allergies, Poor
Disease, Memory loss, Blood Clots, Chronic Infections, Irritable Bowel Syndrome, Chr
Menopause, Herpes Simplex I II, Autoimmune Disorders, Anemia, Eczema, Epstein B
ismitted Diseases, Alcoholism, Tremors, Benign Cysts and Tumors, Drug Addiction,
Depression, Fibrocystic Breast Disease, Chronic Diarrhea, Dermatitis, Hyperthyroid,
Fibroids, Parasites, Pelvic Inflammatory Disease, Panic Attacks, Psoriasis, Lipomas
Candida, Skin Cancer, Rheumatoid Arthritis, Congestive Heart Failure, Kidney Fa
Strokes, Panic Attacks, Hypothyroidism, Lupus, HIV, Kidney Stones, Leukemia, C
evere Burns, Gonorrhea, Schizophrenia, Seizures, Tuberculosis, Lead Poisoning, Pol
Disease, Multiple Sclerosis, Pyelonephritis, Pancreatic Cancer, Ulcerative Colit
ation, Brain Cancer, Juvenile Diabetes, Mitral Valve Prolapse, Syphilis, Crohn's Dise
Addison's Disease, Cirrhosis of the Liver, Scleroderma, Ovarian Cancer, Chlamydia,
sema, Lymphoma, Lou Gehrig's Disease, Gulf War Syndrome, Glaucoma, Liver Can
; Myasthenia Gravis, Trichomonas, Nephrotic Syndrome, Rectal Cancer, Malaria, B
us Sclerosis, Polycystic Kidneys, Muscular Dystrophy, Lyme Disease, Sarcoidosis, Ra
Pituitary Tumors, Galactorrhea, Cystic Fibrosis, Colon Cancer, Parkinson's Disease
ic Fatigue Syndrome, Breast Cancer, Depression, High Blood Pressure, Arthritis, Alzh
e, Asthma, Hepatitis, Cervical Cancer, Coronary Artery Disease, Migraines, Candi
olesterol Endometriosis, Allergies, Poor Circulation, Heart Disease, Memory Loss, Bl
ic Infections, Irritable Bowel Syndrome, Chronic Sinusitis, Menopause, Herpes Simpl
immune Disorders, Anemia, Eczema, Epstein Barr, Sexually Transmitted Diseases, A
ign Cysts, Tumors, Drug Addiction, Infertility, Manic Depression, Fibrocystic Breas
ic Diarrhea, Dermatitis, Hyperthyroidism, Epilepsy, Uterine Fibroids, Parasites, Pe
Disease, Panic Attacks, Psoriasis, Lipomas, Food Allergies, Candida, Skin Cancer,
hritis, Congestive Heart Failure, Kidney Failure, Lung Cancer, Strokes, Panic Attac
lism, Prostate Cancer, Lupus, HIV, Kidney Stones, Leukemia, Chronic Bronchitis, S
rhea, Schizophrenia, Seizures, Tuberculosis, AIDS, Lead Poisoning, Polycystic Ovar
Multiple Sclerosis, Pyelonephritis, Pancreatic Cancer, Ulcerative Colitis, Atrial Fibri
Brain Cancer, Juvenile Diabetes, Mitral Valve Prolapse, Syphilis, Crohn's Disease, C
Addison's Disease, Cirrhosis of the Liver, Emphysema, Scleroderma, Ovarian Cance
lar Degeneration, Retinitis Pigmentosa, Lymphoma, Lou Gehrig's Disease, Gulf Wa
coma, Liver Cancer, Stomach Cancer, Myasthenia Gravis, Trichomonas, Nephrotic
al Cancer, Spinal Cord Injury, Malaria, Birth Defects, Tuberous Sclerosis, Polycysti
ular Dystrophy, Lyme Disease, Sarcoidosis, Raynaud's Disease, Pituitary Tumors, G
Fibrosis, Colon Cancer, Parkinson's Disease, Diabetes, Chronic Fatigue Syndrome, B
ession, High Blood Pressure, Arthritis, Alzheimer's Disease, Asthma, Hepatitis, Cervi
ronary Artery Disease, Migraines, Candida, High Cholesterol Endometriosis, Allerg
lation, Heart Disease, Memory Loss, Blood Clots, Chronic Infections, Irritable Bowe
onic Sinusitis, Menopause, Herpes Simplex I and II, Autoimmune Disorders, Anemi
in Barr, Sexually Transmitted Diseases, Alcoholism, Tremors, Benign Cysts and Tur
ion, Infertility, Cataracts, Macular Degeneration, Manic Depression, Fibrocystic Br
ic Diarrhea, Dermatitis, Hyperthyroidism, Epilepsy, Uterine Fibroids, Parasites, Pe
Disease, Panic Attacks, Psoriasis, Lipomas, Food Allergies, Candida, Skin Cancer,
hritis, Congestive Heart Failure, Kidney Failure, Lung Cancer, Strokes, Fibromyalg
lism, Prostate Cancer, Lupus, HIV, Kidney Stones, Leukemia, Chronic Bronchitis, S
rhea, Schizophrenia, Seizures, Tuberculosis, AIDS, Lead Poisoning, Polycystic Ovar

CHAPTER 4

THE INTESTINAL DETOXIFICATION PROGRAM

The first step in any health program, especially a cleansing or detoxification program, is to stimulate the bowel and cleanse old, toxic material out of the colon.

When you do any type of fast, flush, cleanse or detox, the whole idea is to melt, dissolve and remove toxins and toxic buildup from your fat cells, muscle tissues and organs. When you dissolve this toxic material, it is mostly eliminated from your body by your colon, also called your bowel or large intestine. If your bowel is typical of most Americans', it is slow, sluggish, sleepy and contains pounds of old fecal matter. If you don't stimulate and cleanse your bowel, the poisons that you try to flush out of your body during a cleanse just sit in your intestines and can even be reabsorbed back into your body ALL AT ONCE. This will make you feel awful at best, or could even make you really sick.

So again, the first step is to STIMULATE the colon and REMOVE any old, built up fecal matter.

I spent many years in my clinic developing and perfecting herbal bowel formulae that would cleanse and detoxify the intestinal system. These are powerful herbal formulae that work.

> **"The main function of the body is to repair and heal itself."**
> **– Dr. Richard Schulze**

INTESTINAL CORRECTIVE FORMULA #1

(Cathartic Formula)

Contains: Curacao and Cape Aloe leaf, Senna leaves and pods, Cascara Sagrada aged bark, Barberry rootbark, Ginger rhizome, Garlic bulb and African Bird Pepper.

Therapeutic Action: This stimulating tonic is cleansing, healing and strengthening to the entire gastro-intestinal system. It stimulates your peristaltic action (the muscular movement of the colon) and over time strengthens the muscles of the large intestine. It halts putrefaction and disinfects, soothes and heals the mucous membrane lining of your entire digestive tract. This herbal tonic improves digestion, relieves gas and cramps, increases the flow of bile which in turn cleans the gall bladder, bile ducts and liver, destroys Candida albicans overgrowth and promotes a healthy intestinal flora. It also destroys and expels intestinal parasites, increases gastro-intestinal circulation and is anti-bacterial, anti-viral and anti-fungal.

Continue to use this formula until you are having at least 1 bowel movement each day for every meal you eat. Between 2 and 4 bowel movements a day is normal. Considering all the disease and death we have because of retained fecal matter, I wouldn't worry about taking too much of this formula.

Patient Type A: The sluggish bowel type. This formula is for 97% of my patients, the ones who need help getting their bowel working more frequently. You must use this herbal formula every day to keep your bowels very active.

Dosage: Start with only 1 capsule of this formula during or just after dinner. This formula works best when taken with food or juice. The next morning you should notice an increase in your bowel action and in the amount of fecal matter that you eliminate. The consistency should also be softer. If you do not notice any difference in your bowel behavior by the next day, or if the difference was not dramatic, then that evening increase your dosage to 2 capsules. You can continue to increase your dosage every evening by one capsule until you notice a dramatic difference in the way your bowel works. There is no limit. Most people need only 2-3 capsules but a few have needed over 30 capsules. It has taken most of us years to create a sluggish bowel, so let's be patient for a few days and increase by only 1 capsule each day.

Patient Type B: The irritated bowel type. This only applies to a small percentage of my patients. These are the exceptions to the rule, those with bowels that move too often, (more than 3 times a day.) This includes those with Colitis, Irritable Bowel Syndrome, Crohn's Disease, etc... If your bowels are irritated, hot or working too frequently, skip this formula and go to Intestinal Corrective Formula #2.

INTESTINAL CORRECTIVE FORMULA #2
(Drawing and Detoxifying Formula)

Contains: Flax seed, Apple Fruit Pectin, Pharmaceutical Grade Bentonite Clay, Psyllium seed and husk, Slippery Elm inner bark, Marshmallow root, Fennel seed and Activated Willow charcoal.

Therapeutic Action: This cleansing and soothing formula is to be used in conjunction with Intestinal Formula #1. This formula is a strong purifier and intestinal vacuum. This formula draws old fecal matter off the walls of your colon and out of any bowel pockets. It will remove poisons, toxins, parasites, heavy metals such as mercury and lead and even remove radioactive material such as strontium 90. This formula will also remove over 3,000 known drug residues. Its mucilaginous properties will soften old hardened fecal matter for easy removal and make it an excellent remedy for inflammation in the intestines such as diverticulitis or irritable bowel. Many patients discovered that this formula also removed their colon polyps. This formula is an antidote for food poisoning and other types of poisoning. I always have it with me when I travel.

Before beginning **Intestinal Corrective Formula #2,** your bowels should be moving at least 3 times a day or at least once for each meal you eat. Continue using **Intestinal Corrective Formula #1** until this is achieved.

Dosage: Intestinal Corrective Formula #2 is a drawing and detoxifying formula and will be used at least during weeks 2 and 4 if not all 4 weeks. If you have a serious illness or any intestinal diseases – even polyps or diverticulosuos, do this formula for the entire 4 weeks.

- Take **Intestinal Corrective Formula #2** five times a day.
- Mix one heaping teaspoon of **Intestinal Corrective Formula #2** powder with 8 ounces of juice or distilled water in a jar with a lid. Shake vigorously and drink immediately. Take anytime during the day, just be sure to allow about 30 minutes before or after meals, juices or taking your tinctures.
- Helpful hint: Put a small amount of water in your jar first. Then add the powder and shake. Then add more water. This keeps the powder from sticking to the jar making it easier to clean.
- This formulae contains bentonite clay and may be binding. **Type A's** may need to increase dosage by one of the **Intestinal Corrective Formulae #1. Type B's** may need to take one **Intestinal Corrective Formulae #1** in the evening if you find you are a little constipated.
- **Minor illnesses:** Consume one jar the 2nd week and one jar the 4th week.
- **Serious diseases:** Consume one jar each week.

...rthritis, Alzheimer's Disease, Asthma, Hepatitis, AIDS, Breast Cancer, Coronar...
...rostate Cancer, Candida, Migraines, High Cholesterol, Endometriosis, Allergies, Poor...
...Disease, Memory loss, Blood Clots, Chronic Infections, Irritable Bowel Syndrome, Ch...
...Menopause, Herpes Simplex I II, Autoimmune Disorders, Anemia, Eczema, Epstein...
...nsmitted Diseases, Alcoholism, Tremors, Benign Cysts and Tumors, Drug Addiction,...
...Depression, Fibrocystic Breast Disease, Chronic Diarrhea, Dermatitis, Hyperthyroid...
...e Fibroids, Parasites, Pelvic Inflammatory Disease, Panic Attacks, Psoriasis, Lipomas...
...Candida, Skin Cancer, Rheumatoid Arthritis, Congestive Heart Failure, Kidney Fa...
...; Strokes, Panic Attacks, Hypothyroidism, Lupus, HIV, Kidney Stones, Leukemia, C...
...Severe Burns, Gonorrhea, Schizophrenia, Seizures, Tuberculosis, Lead Poisoning, Po...
...Disease, Multiple Sclerosis, Pyelonephritis, Pancreatic Cancer, Ulcerative Coli...
...ation, Brain Cancer, Juvenile Diabetes, Mitral Valve Prolapse, Syphilis, Crohn's Dis...
...Addison's Disease, Cirrhosis of the Liver, Scleroderma, Ovarian Cancer, Chlamydia...
...sema, Lymphoma, Lou Gehrig's Disease, Gulf War Syndrome, Glaucoma, Liver Can...
...; Myasthenia Gravis, Trichomonas, Nephrotic Syndrome, Rectal Cancer, Malaria, ...
...ous Sclerosis, Polycystic Kidneys, Muscular Dystrophy, Lyme Disease, Sarcoidosis, Ra...
...Pituitary Tumors, Galactorrhea, Cystic Fibrosis, Colon Cancer, Parkinson's Disease...
...ic Fatigue Syndrome, Breast Cancer, Depression, High Blood Pressure, Arthritis, Alzh...
...se, Asthma, Hepatitis, Cervical Cancer, Coronary Artery Disease, Migraines, Candi...
...olesterol Endometriosis, Allergies, Poor Circulation, Heart Disease, Memory Loss, Bl...
...ic Infections, Irritable Bowel Syndrome, Chronic Sinusitis, Menopause, Herpes Simp...
...immune Disorders, Anemia, Eczema, Epstein Barr, Sexually Transmitted Diseases, ...
...ign Cysts, Tumors, Drug Addiction, Infertility, Manic Depression, Fibrocystic Breas...
...ic Diarrhea, Dermatitis, Hyperthyroidism, Epilepsy, Uterine Fibroids, Parasites, Pe...
...e Disease, Panic Attacks, Psoriasis, Lipomas, Food Allergies, Candida, Skin Cancer,...
...hritis, Congestive Heart Failure, Kidney Failure, Lung Cancer, Strokes, Panic Attac...
...dism, Prostate Cancer, Lupus, HIV, Kidney Stones, Leukemia, Chronic Bronchitis, S...
...rrhea, Schizophrenia, Seizures, Tuberculosis, AIDS, Lead Poisoning, Polycystic Ovar...
...Multiple Sclerosis, Pyelonephritis, Pancreatic Cancer, Ulcerative Colitis, Atrial Fibri...
...Brain Cancer, Juvenile Diabetes, Mitral Valve Prolapse, Syphilis, Crohn's Disease, C...
...Addison's Disease, Cirrhosis of the Liver, Emphysema, Scleroderma, Ovarian Cance...
...lar Degeneration, Retinitis Pigmentosa, Lymphoma, Lou Gehrig's Disease, Gulf War...
...ucoma, Liver Cancer, Stomach Cancer, Myasthenia Gravis, Trichomonas, Nephrotic...
...al Cancer, Spinal Cord Injury, Malaria, Birth Defects, Tuberous Sclerosis, Polycysti...
...ular Dystrophy, Lyme Disease, Sarcoidosis, Raynaud's Disease, Pituitary Tumors, G...
...Fibrosis, Colon Cancer, Parkinson's Disease, Diabetes, Chronic Fatigue Syndrome, B...
...ession, High Blood Pressure, Arthritis, Alzheimer's Disease, Asthma, Hepatitis, Cervi...
...ronary Artery Disease, Migraines, Candida, High Cholesterol Endometriosis, Allerg...
...lation, Heart Disease, Memory Loss, Blood Clots, Chronic Infections, Irritable Bowe...
...nic Sinusitis, Menopause, Herpes Simplex I and II, Autoimmune Disorders, Anemia...
...in Barr, Sexually Transmitted Diseases, Alcoholism, Tremors, Benign Cysts and Tu...
...ion, Infertility, Cataracts, Macular Degeneration, Manic Depression, Fibrocystic Br...
...ic Diarrhea, Dermatitis, Hyperthyroidism, Epilepsy, Uterine Fibroids, Parasites, Pe...
...e Disease, Panic Attacks, Psoriasis, Lipomas, Food Allergies, Candida, Skin Cancer,...
...hritis, Congestive Heart Failure, Kidney Failure, Lung Cancer, Strokes, Fibromyalg...
...dism, Prostate Cancer, Lupus, HIV, Kidney Stones, Leukemia, Chronic Bronchitis, S...
...rrhea, Schizophrenia, Seizures, Tuberculosis, AIDS, Lead Poisoning, Polycystic Ovar...

CHAPTER 5

FLUSHES AND ADDITIONAL HERBAL FORMULAE

4 WEEK SCHEDULE

☐ YES
■ NO

	WEEK 1	WEEK 2	WEEK 3	WEEK 4
Liver/Gall Bladder Flush:	YES	NO	YES	NO
D-Tox Formula:	YES	NO	YES	NO
Kidney/Bladder Flush:	NO	YES	NO	YES
Echinacea Plus:	NO	YES	NO	YES

THE LIVER/GALL BLADDER FLUSH DRINK
(1st and 3rd Weeks)

Mix the following in a blender:
- **During Spring or Summer,** mix 8 ounces of fresh orange juice or citrus juice combination (1 lemon or 1 lime and enough orange, grapefruit or tangerine juice to make 8 ounces) or...**During Fall or Winter,** mix 8 ounces of fresh apple and/or grape juice with...
- 8 ounces of distilled or purified water
- 1-5 cloves of garlic (start with 1 clove and increase daily)
- 1-5 tablespoons of organic virgin cold-pressed olive oil (start with 1 tablespoon and increase daily)
- 1 piece of ginger root (about 1 inch long)

15 minutes after this drink, consume 2 cups of **Detoxification Herb Tea** and 2 dropperfuls of **Liver/Gall Bladder & Anti-Parasite Formula.** The **Liver/Gall Bladder & Anti-Parasite Formula** can be taken straight, added to the **Detoxification Herb Tea** or in a few ounces of distilled or purified water. Repeat the **Detoxification Herb Tea** and **Liver/Gall Bladder & Anti-Parasite Formula** 2 more times during the day.

THE KIDNEY/BLADDER FLUSH DRINK
(2nd and 4th Weeks)

Mix the following in a blender:
- Juice of 1 lemon and 1 lime
- 16-32 ounces of distilled or purified water
- A pinch of **Cayenne Powder** or 5-20 drops of **Cayenne Tincture**
- Optional: A small amount of maple syrup to taste

15 minutes after this drink consume 2 cups of **Kidney/Bladder Herb**

Tea and 2 dropperfuls of **Kidney/Bladder Formula.** The **Kidney/Bladder Formula** can be taken straight or added to the **Kidney/Bladder Tea** or in a few ounces of water. Repeat the **Kidney/Bladder Herb Tea** and the **Kidney/Bladder Formula** 2 more times during the day.

ADDITIONAL HERBAL FORMULAE

LIVER/GALL BLADDER & ANTI-PARASITE FORMULA

Contains: Milk Thistle seed, Dandelion root and leaf, Oregon Grape root, Gentian root, Wormwood leaf and flower, Black Walnut hulls, Ginger rhizome, Garlic bulb and Sweet Fennel seed.

Therapeutic Action: The herbs in this formulae are famous for their ability to stimulate, cleanse and protect the liver and gall bladder and rid the body of parasites. Milk Thistle has certain chemicals that bind to and coat liver cells. These phyto-chemicals not only heal previous liver damage but also reduces liver inflammation and protect the liver from future damage. Oregon Grape rootbark, Gentian root, Wormwood leaves and Dandelion root are all classic bitter liver tonic herbs. These herbs not only stimulate digestion but also stimulate the liver to excrete more bile which in turn cleans both the liver and gall bladder. If you have been exposed to any toxic substances, had constipation, eaten large amounts of animal food or drunk alcohol or other harmful beverages this formula is for you. It is also beneficial if you have had high cholesterol, blood fats or any family history of liver or gall bladder problems. Many believe that anyone who has cancer or any immune dysfunction had a weak congested liver to begin with. Even if a person has had their gall bladder removed these herbs will still be effective to clean the liver and bile ducts. The Black Walnut hulls, Wormwood and Garlic are strong ANTI-PARASITICAL plants. Parasite infestation is a fact of life. One cubic inch of beef can have over 1,000 living parasite larvae waiting to hatch in your body. Over 65% of fresh fish tested has toxic levels of bacteria and parasites. Chicken is even worse. I've had hundreds of patients expel bowls full of intestinal parasites, tape worms over 30 FEET LONG and also kill cellular parasites with these formulae. It works best if used in conjunction with both Intestinal Formula #1 and #2. Use if parasites are suspected, or if there has been a history of bowel problems, constipation, eating of animal products, prolonged illness, disease or degeneration.

Dosage: 2 dropperfuls (70 drops) 3 times daily during the 1st and 3rd weeks of the 30-Day Program. Most effective if used in conjunction with the next formula, the Detoxification Herb Tea.

DETOXIFICATION HERB TEA

Contains: Roasted Dandelion root, Burdock root, Pau d' Arco inner bark, Cinnamon bark, Cardamon seed, Licorice root, Fennel seed, Juniper berries, Ginger root, Clove buds, Black Peppercorns, Uva Ursi leaves, Horsetail herb, Orange peel and Parsley root.

Therapeutic Action: This tea has numerous health benefits. First, it is based on an ancient East Indian digestive tea formula. Over the years in my clinic I saw my patients eat almost anything and survive if they drank a cup of this tea before, during and after the meal. It stimulates the entire digestive process, especially the stomach during the first stages of digestion.

This tea also cleanses the blood, skin, liver and gall bladder and is the perfect tea to use after the liver flush. It flushes out the bile and fats that the liver flush purged from your liver and gall bladder. It is also a mild diuretic and disinfectant to the kidneys and bladder and will cause you to urinate a little more within an hour after ingestion.

This tea is also an excellent coffee replacement. It is a hot beverage, dark in color and tastes good. It's even better when a little pure maple syrup is added to the final brew. It also increases your circulation but has no caffeine. I used it in my clinic successfully for years to help people get off the coffee habit.

Dosage: Drink 2 cups of the tea 15 minutes after doing your Liver/Gall Bladder Flush. It can also be drunk at any other time during the day, as many cups as desired. Drink 2 cups 2 more times during the day. Put 1 tablespoon (medium) or 2 tablespoons (strong) of this tea into 20 ounces of distilled water. Be sure to use only stainless steel or glass cookware. Let the tea sit in the water overnight. In the morning heat to a boil, reduce heat and let simmer for 15 minutes. Strain the herbs, but do not discard them. Let tea cool a bit, but drink hot. Put the used herbs back into the pot, adding 1 tablespoon of fresh herbs and 20 ounces of distilled water. Let sit overnight and repeat whole process again. Keep adding new herbs to old ones for 3 days, then discard all herbs and start over.

KIDNEY/BLADDER FORMULA

Contains: Uva Ursi leaves, Juniper berries, Corn silk, Horsetail herb, Pipsissewa leaf, Burdock root and seed and Goldenrod flower tops.

Therapeutic Action: This tonic is both diuretic (increases the flow of urine) and disinfectant to the kidneys, bladder and urinary system. According to medical reports the herbs in this formula destroy the bacteria that cause kidney and bladder infections. More importantly, whenever I used these formulae in my clinic, it cured every patient with a urinary tract infection, even after antibiotics had failed. It worked 100% of the time. This tonic formula works best if used along with the Kidney/Bladder Tea and the Kidney/Bladder Flush.

Dosage: 2 dropperfuls (70 drops) 3 times daily during the 2nd and 4th weeks of the 30-Day Program. Best results are obtained if used along with the Kidney/Bladder Herb Tea.

KIDNEY/BLADDER & DISSOLVE TEA FORMULA

Contains: Juniper berries, Corn silk, Uva Ursi leaves, Parsley root and leaf, Carrot tops, Dandelion leaf, Horsetail herb, Goldenrod flower tops, Hydrangea root, Gravel root and Marshmallow root, Orange peel and Peppermint leaf.

Therapeutic Action: Same powerful effect as the Kidney/Bladder Formula above. This tea is most effective if used along with the tonic. This formula also completely dissolves stubborn kidney stones and calculi.

Dosage: 2 cups 3 times daily.

THE D-TOX FORMULA

Contains: Red Clover blossoms, Mojave Chaparral herb and resin, Poke root, Oregon Grape root, Burdock root and seed, Yellow Dock root, Goldenseal root, Bloodroot, Garlic Juice, Lobelia seeds and Cayenne.

Therapeutic Action: This is a very powerful blood and lymph cleansing formula and the one that I've used for years in my clinic. These herbs are famous for scrubbing the accumulated toxins and poisons out of the body's blood, fat and cells. Every patient that did the 30-Day Program consumes 1 bottle of this formula during the 2nd and 4th weeks. Chaparral is one of nature's most powerful anti-oxidants and has proven itself in the clinic to break-up, destroy and dissolve all types of tumors. The herbs in this formula are strong in taste, and very effective detoxifiers. Every patient I saw with chronic illness or degeneration used this formula with great success.

Dosage: Take 2 dropperfuls (70 drops) 5 times a day. Consume 1 entire bottle the 1st week and 1 entire bottle the 3rd week, alternating the 2nd and 4th weeks with **Echinacea Plus.**

ECHINACEA PLUS

Contains: Fresh Echinacea angustifolia root JUICE, Echinacea angustifolia root, Echinacea purpurea seed, Fresh Garlic bulb juice and Habanero pepper.

Therapeutic Action: Echinacea is one of the strongest immune stimulators and enhancers known. It can double and triple the amount of T-cells and Macrophages in your bloodstream within a few days. It can also increase the amount of Interferon, Interleukin, Immunoglobulin and other important natural immune chemicals present in your blood. This is how Echinacea works, by boosting the number of immune cells and the amount of natural immune chemicals, then stimulating them into more activity. The benefit of immune stimulation is a shorter duration of existing colds and flu and/or prevention of future infections. It also initiates and speeds up recovery from chronic and long-term immune-related depression illnesses, diseases and degeneration.
Cayenne is the best herb to stimulate circulation and makes these already powerful immune herbs many times more effective. Garlic is the best, most effective broad spectrum antibiotic, anti-viral, anti-fungal herb known. Echinacea, Garlic and Cayenne are a Dynamic Herbal Trio.

Dosage: Take 2 dropperfuls (70 drops) 5 times a day. You should consume one entire bottle of **Echinacea Plus** the 2nd week, and one entire bottle the 4th week, alternating weeks 1 and 3 with the **D-Tox Formula.**

CAYENNE TINCTURE

Contains: FRESH JUICE of Organic Habanero peppers, California Jalapeno, African Bird Peppers, Chinese, Korean, Thai and Japanese peppers.

Therapeutic Action: Cayenne is the greatest herbal aid to circulation and can be used on a regular basis. The extract is VERY concentrated and gets in the bloodstream fast which makes it a perfect first aid remedy, for heart attacks, stroke, fainting, shock, dizziness, internal or external bleeding. Use a few drops to 10 dropperfuls. It has saved many lives.

Dosage: 5 to 30 drops 3 times daily, CAUTION extremely HOT. During this 30-Day Program you will have moments that you feel a lull or are even exhausted. Cayenne will bring you back to life fast. A few drops of the tincture put directly into your mouth or a few dropperfuls in a small glass of water will do the trick. It will stimulate your circulation, if not blow your head off.

If you are doing the Intensive version of the 30-Day Program, **Cayenne Tincture** is even more important. If you are feeling weak, faint or are going to pass out during the Cold Sheet Treatment, immediately take a dropperful of **Cayenne Tincture** directly into your mouth. Now try and pass out. I dare you.

Cayenne has many first aid applications and can do many things but waking you up and keeping you conscious is what we are talking about here.

DR. SCHULZE'S SPECIAL BLEND OF CAYENNE POWDER

Contains: A special blend of California, Florida and Mexican Habanero Peppers, African Birdeye Peppers, Chinese Hot Reds, Korean Aji, Thai Red, Japanese Red, California Jalapeno's and Serrano's.

This formula is a serious blend of the hottest cayenne peppers in the world. The peppers I use range in heat units from 90,000 to 575,000. You read it right, 575,000! No one else uses peppers in this heat range, if they could even find them. When I mix it, I have to wear a special gas mask that I bought from the German Special Forces. I am NOT kidding!

Therapeutic Action: The benefits of daily cayenne usage are widely known. It is the greatest circulation stimulant known.

Dosage: CAUTION, start with a small amount! **DO NOT** encapsulate. Put a small amount in a little juice, stir and chug. Work your way up in dosage slowly. 1/8 to 1/2 teaspoon 2 to 4 times daily.

LOBELIA TINCTURE

Contains: Lobelia seeds in Organic Raw Apple Cider Vinegar and pure Grain Alcohol

Therapeutic Action: Lobelia is one of the most powerful and versatile herbs I know of. In my clinic I learned to rely on this herb more than any other.

Lobelia has two main uses. First, as an antispasmodic, it is second to none and will relax the entire body and organs. On a milder level you may be so energetically high from your 30-Day Program that you may find you need a lot less sleep. When it's time, Lobelia will bring you down. Some people who are more ill may have spasms, cramps, even fits and convulsions. Lobelia will stop them in seconds. Just put a whole dropperful into their mouth and the body will calm right down.

Secondly, Lobelia is also the greatest herb for lung problems. IT IS A STRONG BRONCHIAL DILATOR. It will get you breathing easily again. It also will help you to expectorate material out of the lungs. I have seen it work with a hundred different disorders.

Dosage: 5 to 60 drops 3 to 4 times daily. In an emergency, use 2 to 5 dropperfuls or more. An overdose is not dangerous, but causes sweating and nausea.

Cayenne Tincture cranks things up and **Lobelia Tincture** brings things down. You should never be without these two herbs in case of an emergency. Keep them in your pocket, in your car, and in your desk at the office. ALWAYS HAVE THESE TWO HERBS ON HAND, especially during this 30-Day Program. Tinctures are herbal liquid extracts. They are the best because they are easy to use and fast acting. (Just squirt into your mouth.) They are more concentrated than teas, get into your bloodstream immediately and have a shelf life of forever.

ostate Cancer, Candida, Migraines, High Cholesterol, Endometriosis, Allergies, Poor
Disease, Memory loss, Blood Clots, Chronic Infections, Irritable Bowel Syndrome, Ch
Menopause, Herpes Simplex I II, Autoimmune Disorders, Anemia, Eczema, Epstein B
smitted Diseases, Alcoholism, Tremors, Benign Cysts and Tumors, Drug Addiction,
Depression, Fibrocystic Breast Disease, Chronic Diarrhea, Dermatitis, Hyperthyroidi
Fibroids, Parasites, Pelvic Inflammatory Disease, Panic Attacks, Psoriasis, Lipomas,
Candida, Skin Cancer, Rheumatoid Arthritis, Congestive Heart Failure, Kidney Fai
Strokes, Panic Attacks, Hypothyroidism, Lupus, HIV, Kidney Stones, Leukemia, Cl
evere Burns, Gonorrhea, Schizophrenia, Seizures, Tuberculosis, Lead Poisoning, Pol
Disease, Multiple Sclerosis, Pyelonephritis, Pancreatic Cancer, Ulcerative Coliti
tion, Brain Cancer, Juvenile Diabetes, Mitral Valve Prolapse, Syphilis, Crohn's Dise
Addison's Disease, Cirrhosis of the Liver, Scleroderma, Ovarian Cancer, Chlamydia,
ema, Lymphoma, Lou Gehrig's Disease, Gulf War Syndrome, Glaucoma, Liver Canc
Myasthenia Gravis, Trichomonas, Nephrotic Syndrome, Rectal Cancer, Malaria, B
us Sclerosis, Polycystic Kidneys, Muscular Dystrophy, Lyme Disease, Sarcoidosis, Ray
Pituitary Tumors, Galactorrhea, Cystic Fibrosis, Colon Cancer, Parkinson's Disease,
c Fatigue Syndrome, Breast Cancer, Depression, High Blood Pressure, Arthritis, Alzhe
, Asthma, Hepatitis, Cervical Cancer, Coronary Artery Disease, Migraines, Candid
esterol Endometriosis, Allergies, Poor Circulation, Heart Disease, Memory Loss, Blo
c Infections, Irritable Bowel Syndrome, Chronic Sinusitis, Menopause, Herpes Simple
nmune Disorders, Anemia, Eczema, Epstein Barr, Sexually Transmitted Diseases, A
gn Cysts, Tumors, Drug Addiction, Infertility, Manic Depression, Fibrocystic Breast
c Diarrhea, Dermatitis, Hyperthyroidism, Epilepsy, Uterine Fibroids, Parasites, Pel
Disease, Panic Attacks, Psoriasis, Lipomas, Food Allergies, Candida, Skin Cancer, F
ritis, Congestive Heart Failure, Kidney Failure, Lung Cancer, Strokes, Panic Attack
ism, Prostate Cancer, Lupus, HIV, Kidney Stones, Leukemia, Chronic Bronchitis, Se
hea, Schizophrenia, Seizures, Tuberculosis, AIDS, Lead Poisoning, Polycystic Ovari
ultiple Sclerosis, Pyelonephritis, Pancreatic Cancer, Ulcerative Colitis, Atrial Fibrill
rain Cancer, Juvenile Diabetes, Mitral Valve Prolapse, Syphilis, Crohn's Disease, Ch
ddison's Disease, Cirrhosis of the Liver, Emphysema, Scleroderma, Ovarian Cancer,
r Degeneration, Retinitis Pigmentosa, Lymphoma, Lou Gehrig's Disease, Gulf War
oma, Liver Cancer, Stomach Cancer, Myasthenia Gravis, Trichomonas, Nephrotic S
l Cancer, Spinal Cord Injury, Malaria, Birth Defects, Tuberous Sclerosis, Polycystic
ar Dystrophy, Lyme Disease, Sarcoidosis, Raynaud's Disease, Pituitary Tumors, Ga
ibrosis, Colon Cancer, Parkinson's Disease, Diabetes, Chronic Fatigue Syndrome, Bre
ssion, High Blood Pressure, Arthritis, Alzheimer's Disease, Asthma, Hepatitis, Cervic
onary Artery Disease, Migraines, Candida, High Cholesterol Endometriosis, Allergie
ation, Heart Disease, Memory Loss, Blood Clots, Chronic Infections, Irritable Bowel
ic Sinusitis, Menopause, Herpes Simplex I and II, Autoimmune Disorders, Anemia,
n Barr, Sexually Transmitted Diseases, Alcoholism, Tremors, Benign Cysts and Tum
n, Infertility, Cataracts, Macular Degeneration, Manic Depression, Fibrocystic Bre
c Diarrhea, Dermatitis, Hyperthyroidism, Epilepsy, Uterine Fibroids, Parasites, Pel
Disease, Panic Attacks, Psoriasis, Lipomas, Food Allergies, Candida, Skin Cancer, F
ritis, Congestive Heart Failure, Kidney Failure, Lung Cancer, Strokes, Fibromyalgia
ism, Prostate Cancer, Lupus, HIV, Kidney Stones, Leukemia, Chronic Bronchitis, Se
hea, Schizophrenia, Seizures, Tuberculosis, AIDS, Lead Poisoning, Polycystic Ovari
Sclerosis, Pyelonephritis, Pancreatic Cancer, Ulcerative Coliti, Atrial Fibrilla

CHAPTER 6

HYDROTHERAPY

THE POWER OF HYDROTHERAPY

Blockage - The Cause of all Disease

After my first few years in clinical practice, it became obvious to me that wherever I saw a disease, any disease, that area of the body had been blocked off from the rest of the body in some way. There can be blockages of blood flow, preventing blood that brings oxygen and nutrients that your cells need to re-build themselves and create health, or there can be blockages of the lymphatic flow. The lymphatic flow brings immune cells to sick areas to heal them, and also removes waste material from the cells. There can also be blockages in nerve flow or nerve force to the area. There can be blockages of what the Chinese call "Chi" or what the Japanese call "Ki" or what the Indians call "Prana" or "life energy." There can be muscular spasms cutting off all types of circulation. There can even be emotional or spiritual blockage to an area – not enough love moving in, and too much hate and rage building up. If there is one thing I know for sure; **Every sick area of the body has some type of physical, emotional or spiritual blockage.**

After 20 years of clinical practice, exploring numerous therapies, nothing broke up blockage and drove blood and life back into a blocked, diseased area faster or better than Hot and Cold Hydrotherapy.

> **"All disease is caused by some type of blockage, whether it's lymphatic, digestive, nutritional, elimination, emotional, whatever. Free the blockage, let the energy flow and healing begins immediately."**
> **– Dr. Richard Schulze**

A Brief History of Hydrotherapy

As far back as any recorded medical or scientific history, even back to ancient Mesopotamia, India, Egypt and China, there have been records of people using hot and cold water to cure. These therapies go back five or six thousand years. In 18th Century Europe, there were numerous people who found that hydrotherapy healed disease - especially those that no doctor, either natural or even the new medicine, was able to help. It became a big part of European natural therapy to use hot and cold applications. By the 19th Century, the use of hydrotherapy spread throughout Europe and America. Hydrotherapy centers were set up all over the world from Malverne, England to Spa, Belgium to Baaden, Germany to Hot Springs, Arkansas. All these centers were famous for curing the "incurables" and healing diseases that no other form of therapy could. A great European natural doctor named Dr. Benedict Lust even developed a treatment called the "Blood Washing Method," and wrote a book on it by the same name. It was an eight-hour treatment – a constant eight hours of hydrotherapy. It was mainly a cold shower for eight hours. So if anybody thinks that I've gone over the top here, my program would be considered lightweight to middle-of-the-road in any of the 19th century hydrotherapy clinics. Some of these clinics would literally strap you to the wall and hit you with an ice cold fire hose. This may sound radical but not compared to surgery, chemotherapy and radiation.

The Power of Hot and Cold and How It Works

There are a lot of different ways to increase circulation to an area that's blocked off and diseased. There are herbs that you can take that will increase your blood flow – powerful herbs like cayenne and ginger. There are herbs that you can use that will thin your blood like garlic. Garlic will even thin the lymphatic fluid, which will help the lymphatic flow. There's lymphatic massage. There are all types of Swedish massage, which will help move the fluids in your body. Massage/bodywork, exercise, yoga – these will all help release the muscles and help stimulate the nervous system. There are foods for the nerves and foods for the muscles. There are meditations, mantras and positive affirmations you can do that will heal the emotional blockages. There are prayers for the spiritual blockages. Of all these routines put together, the one that I saw in my clinic that was the fastest and most powerful way to move blood in and out of an area was the application of hot and cold.

Hot Water

Hot water, or anything that's hot, when applied to the surface of the body, dilates the capillaries and veins, and draws the blood out of the depths of the body, and up to the surface of the body. It immediately changes your blood flow and brings it all to the surface. Hot therapy also relaxes your muscles, which in turn allows better lymphatic flow, which in turn takes pressure off of nerves and allows better nerve flow. Hot water is also physically and emotionally sedating. So here you have an application that brings the blood to the surface of the body and increases the blood flow. It sedates you and relaxes the muscles, which allows the lymph and the nervous systems to flow better.

Cold Water

When you apply cold water to the surface of the body, it has exactly the opposite effect. It contracts the capillaries and veins on the surface of the body and drives the blood deep into the center of your body. So it moves the blood in the exact opposite direction. It contracts the muscles which in turn pushes the lymphatic fluid out of the area. This is also a massage for the nerves. It is the opposite of sedating. It is exciting, and invigorating. It wakes you up. On a physical and emotional level, it has the opposite effect of the application of heat.

Hot and Cold

You can use hot water to relax yourself in a bath or cold water to wake you up in a shower, but what we're talking about here is healing disease with Hydrotherapy. One of the greatest ways to stimulate a blocked area and heal disease is to get the blood to flow in and out of that area *rapidly*, to get the lymphatic fluid to flow in and out of that area *rapidly*, to contract the muscles and relax the muscles *rapidly*, to stimulate the nervous system and to sedate the nervous system *rapidly*, to wake you up and put you back to sleep *rapidly*. This is not only the strongest way to move the blood; it is the strongest way to move the lymph, to stimulate the nerves, to tone the muscles and to affect you emotionally. This treatment of hot and cold is more powerful than that of any herb or treatment from Cayenne to Psychotherapy. I saw this treatment literally move mountains.

THE HOT AND COLD SHOWER ROUTINE

Frequency: Everyone - 1-3 times per day.

In my clinic, I developed the Hot and Cold Shower Routine to stimulate blood flow in and out of an area and heal it. My patients would use this for anything from a bruise to an injured hip, all the way to tumors in breast cancer.

This routine is simple.

While taking a nice, warm shower, turn up the hot water until it's as hot as you can stand it, making sure the hot water is hitting the area that is blocked or injured. When you've had the hot water on the area for about a minute, turn it off completely so that you have straight, cold water hitting the area. Let the cold water hit the area for 15-30 seconds. Now, it will be a shock. That's okay. If you need to shake - Shake! If you need to cry – Cry! If you need to scream – Scream! And if you need to pee yourself – Hey, you're in the shower. I'm always leery of anyone who can do a hot and cold shower without letting out a squeak. Let it out! Once the area is thoroughly cold after about thirty seconds, turn the hot water back up slowly until the hot water is as hot as you can stand it and leave it on that area for a minute. Once that area is hot for a minute, turn the hot water off quickly and turn the cold water on fully. The point is to shock your body. Repeat the hot and cold seven times. In the morning end with cold to stimulate you and wake you up. In the evening, end with hot to sedate and relax you. The procedure will only take between 10 and 15 minutes, but you will feel like a new person when it's over. You can repeat this Hot and Cold Shower Routine again the same day or do a partial one just applying hot and cold water directly to the affected area.

While doing this Hot and Cold Shower Routine, make sure to pay special attention to the affected area and massage that area vigorously. If the shower is impossible, use your imagination. You may need to be sitting in hot and cold buckets. Use hot packs and ice packs if you need to. Many times, if you'll do this routine within 10 minutes of being injured, you will have no more soreness, pain or even bruising . If you have a degenerative disease like a breast cancer, you would do this hot and cold shower routine three times a day and of course add massage and skin brushing over the breast area. Don't underestimate the power of this simple, Hot and Cold Shower Routine.

Case History
I had a man with melanoma (skin cancer) with a large spot on his back. He did my 30-Day Program for 2 months and felt a lot better, but there was no change in the skin cancer. In talking to him, I found out that he did not do the hot and cold therapy on his back because he just felt that he couldn't take it, that it would be too intense. I explained to him that he did not do *my* 30-Day Program but that he did *his* version of it. Often the part of the program that a person skips is the part they need the most.

I told him that he needed to go back and begin the program again, this time not leaving out the Hot and Cold Shower Routines. Within three days, he called and told me that by adding the hot and cold showers, that the skin cancer on his back fell off in the middle of his Hot and Cold Shower Routine. It actually just fell off his body.

HOW TO DO A HIGH ENEMA

Frequency:
- Everyone: 1 time every other week
- Minor illness: 1-2 times per week
- Serious, killer disease: 2-3 times per week.

A high enema is designed to wash, empty and clean out the entire colon, and large intestines. By comparison, a regular enema only washes fecal matter out of the area near your rectum. In addition, a high enema should always be followed by a rectal implant.

You can do a high enema at home. It's easy. The first time you have to be patient. I always say it's best to have an enema party. It's much easier if you have two people – one person giving the enema and one person receiving. Otherwise, you've got to work and move and strain all on your own.

Put a couple of old towels down on your bathroom floor because chances are you are going to get a little bit of water on the floor, possibly a little bit of fecal matter, some herbal ointment and other things. Make it nice and comfortable. Put a heater in the bathroom and get it warmed up. Play some nice, enema music and spray some essential oil or light some incense because you'll have old fecal matter coming out and this is going to smell. So make it a nice experience.

Make sure you apply some herbal ointment or un-petroleum jelly. Grease your rectum really well. You are better off over-greased than under-greased. Fill the enema bag with nice, warm water – body temperature or a little cooler. If you are prone to having your bowel be a little spastic, you can add 1/2-1 dropperful of **Lobelia Tincture**.

Begin with a regular enema. While lying on the floor, release the clamp and let the air out of the tube before introducing the water. Have your healing partner introduce 8-16 ounces of water into your rectum. At this point, many people will feel an initial cramp like, "Oh, I gotta get this out of here now." So hop on the toilet and let that water and fecal matter out of the bowel. And do that again. You can repeat a rectal flush two or three times. After a while, just water comes out.

Now you want to introduce water into the colon itself, and it's very simple. First, lie on your left side. Have your healing partner put the enema in, and refill the bag with at least a couple of quarts of water if you can get that much in. Have your healing partner unclip the enema hose so the water starts flowing.

You'll feel the water enter the rectum. Breathe. You need to breathe. Take some deep breaths and relax. You might feel a little cramping. If you do, say, "Stop." Your healing partner will shut off the flow of the enema bag. Have them keep it off for a while until the cramping subsides.

You'll begin to feel the water on your left side, especially if you're using cooler water. You'll begin to feel it entering your sigmoid and descending colon. Again, if you feel a cramp, or, like, "Oh, I can't hold this!" tell your healing partner to stop the water. Relax and breathe, but do try to get as much water in as possible.

There's no hurry to get up. You'll empty your rectum, but you'll also have some emptying of your descending or sigmoid colon. Lie back, use a little more herbal ointment or unpetroleum jelly, fill the enema bag again, and then lie down again on your left side. The second or third time, you'll probably get a lot of water in. In fact, you'll probably drain the enema bag.

You'll feel the water on your left side, all the way up under your rib. This is called your splenic flexure, because it's the bend right near your spleen.

Now, roll over, onto your back. It helps if you put an old pillow under your butt to elevate you a bit. Once on a slant, you'll feel the water enter your transverse colon moving from left to right, going backwards through the colon, the opposite way the fecal matter goes.

Now you'll <u>feel</u> the water, and when you feel it go all the way above your navel at the base of your rib cage through your transverse colon, you may feel as though you have a belly or lower abdomen full of water. It will feel a little heavy. Great!

Now, turn over onto your right side. As you move, you might have to have a water change. Have your healing partner pull the enema out. (In Europe, they have enema bags that have open tops so you can keep adding water as this is going on, but in this country, we have sealed enema bags, so you have to stop, pull out the enema, fill the enema bag again and then restart. If you can, cut a hole in the top of your sealed enema bag so you can refill it without removing the hose from your rectum.) Now you are filling up the right side of your colon. You'll feel that water going down the ascending colon all the way down to that cecum and appendix, which is halfway between your navel and your hip bone.

If you drew a line between your navel and what's called the iliac crest of your pelvis, that's about where your cecum is. You'll feel it all the way there. When you've had enough, stop. Say, "I'm full of water," and lie there. Maybe even get up into a higher slant where your butt is even higher. If you've got support under you, it will help distribute the water.

If you've done yoga, try a shoulder stand or a modified one. If you haven't done yoga, put your feet up against the wall and walk your feet up the wall creating a slight inversion. Stay there and relax.

Be there for at least 5 minutes, if not 10 to 15 minutes. Then get on the toilet. Relax. You may find that, at first, nothing comes out. Then, as you relax more, water will come out and you'll think, "Was that it?"

Relax even more, and you'll have a real flush of water. You'll get a tremendous amount of water and a lot more fecal matter now. When you finish that, if you are up to it, start all over again.

At this point, you won't have to do any more rectal flushes. Your body will accept a high enema immediately. So do it again. You'll find that you can do two or three of these before the water starts looking somewhat clear.

If you're lucky, you'll get what's called a cecal flush, which means you're sitting on the toilet and, all of a sudden, you'll feel a cramp in your bowel. The whole bowel contracts at once and you have a cecal flush. A cecal flush means that the water from your cecum all the way through your bowel is expelled at once. On the way to the toilet, it will feel very warm – even hot, and you'll feel a peristaltic wave from your right side to your left. It's tremendous. Now you know you've done some deep cleansing. In the colonic industry that's called a cecal flush, and if you can get it at home with a high enema, yahoo!

When you're more advanced, you can have your healing partner do some abdominal rocking, putting their hand on your abdomen while you are on your back, and rocking you back and forth. That should relax you. If you are more advanced, you can even have your healing partner do a light massage on your abdomen.

What can be even more beneficial is if your healing partner does foot reflexology on the colon points, or a neck rub. Anything to help you relax. Any type of bodywork works well.

Your high enema must be followed by an implant. Fill your enema bag with one of the following implant formulae. Introduce the implant into your bowel and don't let it out. Just relax and leave it in there, and you'll find it will mostly be absorbed. Your colon absorbs massive amounts of water – that's one of its jobs – to absorb liquid. If you're putting red clover, chaparral, wheat grass juice, or aloe vera in your bowel, these herbs will be absorbed directly into the bowel tissue.

<u>Implant Formulae Options:</u>

1. Soothing: 8 ounces of aloe vera juice and 8 ounces of distilled water

OR

2. Detoxifying: 2 ounces wheatgrass juice with 16 ounces distilled water

OR

3. Use Your Imagination: If you feel you need a blood-cleansing tea as an implant, use red clover, or chaparral, or use echinacea root tea for its immune-enhancing abilities.

The amount of minerals you take out of your colon with an enema is not significant. You can rebuild your body's mineral supply with a small amount of sea vegetable, an almond, or a couple of Brazil nuts. We're not talking about doing an enema every day of your life. If you are really sick, we're talking twice a week until you get well. For those who are not as sick, we're talking once a week or at even greater intervals.

> **"The healing journey you are about to embark on is not a burden or a chore, but a blessing. It will be your greatest adventure inward to discover and create a new life, a new you."**
>
> **– Dr. Richard Schulze**

DR. SCHULZE'S
COLD SHEET TREATMENT

Creating an Artificial Fever

In natural healing we do just the opposite of medicine. We know that fever is the body's way of reacting to an infection or disease. Fever is actually part of the cellular mediated immune response. When your immune cells discover a disease or bacteria in your body, the area naturally becomes hot. One of the reasons it becomes hot is because of the amount of white blood cells that engorge this area. The cells actually excrete chemicals that tell your body to raise its temperature. This is sometimes referred to as leukotaxis. This happens for a number of reasons. For every degree of temperature rise in your body, the speed at which your white cells can travel to the disease and their effectiveness is doubled. What that means is that if you have a 104 degree fever, the speed at which your white blood cells can move is 64 times faster than at a normal temperature of 98 degrees. The point is, the fever is created by the immune system in order to speed up its process of destroying the invader or disease. The last thing we want to do is to suppress a fever. Suppressing a fever impairs the immune system. This is one of the main problems with medicine. People get worse when their fever is suppressed. In natural healing we know that a fever is never dangerous as long as you keep hydrating your body with plenty of liquid. We want to stimulate the fever and in the case of the Cold Sheet Treatment, we want to induce an artificial fever.

Ways To Win On The Cold Sheet Treatment

Whether you're giving yourself an enema or you're giving yourself a Cold Sheet Treatment, you need to have an extremely supportive and positive partner. Get over the embarrassment of the enema because they're going to have their finger in your butt. Get over the embarrassment of being naked because you're curing yourself of a killer disease.

You can't give yourself a Cold Sheet Treatment. We've had a few patients that did and God bless them. So find someone who has the guts to put you through a routine that is very intense. Your chances of being successful in doing a Cold Sheet Treatment and healing yourself are 1,000 times greater if you have a support person to do it with.

I do not suggest that this person be your husband or your wife or the person that you live with unless they are 1,000% supportive of what you're doing. In almost every circumstance, I found it to be better with a friend from the health food store or another student of natural healing – not the person that you live with. In fact, often things come out when you're in the hot tub that you wouldn't want the person you're living with to hear.

The first time you do a new healing procedure, especially the Cold Sheet Treatment, you may have some fear and anxiety. It may be scary because this is all new to you. After the first one, however, you will see that you survived and didn't hurt yourself. After 2 or 3 you will be an expert. As you begin to relax and really get into the program you will start to get the maximum benefit from this powerful treatment.

> **"Trust yourself and stop asking so many questions. You will find your own answers as you go through the process."**
> **– Dr. Richard Schulze**

INSTRUCTIONS ON
THE COLD SHEET TREATMENT

Frequency:
- Minor illness: Once during the 30-day program.
- Terminal illness: Once per week or more.

I have provided a list of supplies you will need. Get everything you need in advance and follow these step-by-step instructions.

Supplies:
- Plastic drop cloths (several)
- Four 100% cotton sheets
- Extra blankets (non-synthetic)
- Several old towels and wash cloths
- Bucket (large enough for 20 pounds of ice and a sheet)
- 20 pounds of ice
- Stainless steel or glass pot to cook tea in
- Old cotton t-shirt and string to tie off (to make large tea bag)
- Enema Bag
- Olive oil (lubricant) or herbal salve or unpetrolium gel
- Blender
- 8 ounces Distilled water
- 8 ounces Organic Apple Cider Vinegar
- Rectal syringe
- Vaseline
- Thermometer (optional)

Herbal Supplies:
- Cayenne Tincture
- Lobelia Tincture
- 1 ounce Cayenne Powder
- Yarrow flower or sage leaf and ginger (to make tea with)

- 8-10 cloves garlic
- 1 ounce Ginger root powder
- 1 ounce Dry Mustard seed powder
- Dr. Schulze's Clinical Air Treatment

1. Cover your bed with plastic before you start the wet part of this program. On top of the plastic, put two 100% cotton sheets.

2. Place the third 100% cotton sheet in the bucket with the 20 pounds of ice. Add about a gallon of water. Make sure the sheet and ice are mixed together well.

3. Brew a pot (6-8 cups) of yarrow, sage or ginger tea. This tea needs to be guzzled, so don't make it too hot. If you don't have or can't find the herbs, hot water with lemon will do.

4. Prepare a hot bath.

Begin filling the bathtub with hot water. This hot water will be sitting for about 10 minutes before you get in.

Make a large tea bag out of your cut up t-shirt. Fill the bag half way to allow room for the herbs to expand. Fill with the following herbs:

- 1 ounce (or a handful) of Cayenne powder
- 1 ounce (or a handful) of Mustard seed powder
- 1 ounce (or a handful) of Ginger root powder

Tightly tie off with cotton string.

Place this tea bag in your bathtub filled with hot, hot water. The water will turn a yellowy orange. Squeeze the bag every so often to activate the herbs. The fumes will choke you a bit. They might even downright gag you because of the volatile oils coming out of the herbs.

If you can't find these herbs in powder form, use whatever form you can find – fresh, dried, etc...

5. Enema

Fill your enema bag with cool, distilled water. If you want, you can take half an hour and do a complete high enema or colonic. At the minimum, you want to empty the rectum of fecal matter.

6. Garlic Injection

You will be using your rectal syringe for this garlic injection. You can find a rectal syringe at your local pharmacy.

Liquefy in a blender:
- 8 ounces distilled water
- 8 ounces organic apple cider vinegar
- 6-10 cloves of garlic

Put liquid mixture in rectal syringe. Lubricate the rectum and the end of the rectal syringe with olive oil. Insert the syringe without squeezing the bulb. Take a few deep breaths, then squeeze the bulb. Try to get this mixture in all at once. You will not get a second chance, because it will want to come right back out. Stay close to the toilet. This will burn, and you will want to evacuate it quickly. It will take you about 2 minutes to recover, then you can move on to the next step.

7. Hot Bath

Important: Before you get in this hot, herbal bath you must cover your **genitals, anus, nipples and any extra sensitive areas or wounds** with plenty of Vaseline to protect them. Herbal oils will not work. **Don't forget this step!**

We know that Vaseline is a petroleum product, but having your genitals on fire could ruin this treatment.

20-30 minutes is your goal. This is when you will need a committed healing partner, someone that will push you that extra inch. It may be that extra inch that will heal you.

Enter the bathtub, start running more hot water into the tub. You want the water to be as hot as you can stand it. Breathe! Breathe! Scream and holler if you have to, **but stay in the tub.**

Begin to **consume your 6-7 cups of tea.** It is very important to drink lots of liquid while in the hot bathtub. You do not need to worry about dehydration due to your fever if you are consuming lots of tea.

Force the tea down. You have only 15-20 minutes in this tub. Your healing partner should have your next cup of tea ready before you finish the current one. The point is, you must drink the tea quickly. No sipping! If you throw up a little, that's OK. Just keep drinking.

Keep your Cayenne Tincture close by in case you get light-headed and feel like you are going to faint. Use the Lobelia Tincture if you are having any kind of spasm.

The first 5-10 minutes, you won't feel anything unusual. Then you will begin to feel an uncomfortable burning sensation. Very soon after this, you will say you have had enough, that you have had it and you are on fire. At this point, you must stay in 5 more minutes. In the last 5 minutes is when all the physical and emotional healing takes place. Crying, sobbing, screaming, hysteria and hallucinations are common. Experience it all. Let it all out as the old saying goes. But don't get out of that tub. Breathe!

I have never, ever seen these herbs burn anyone's skin. It will only feel like it. Your breaking point is way beyond what you think it is. Breathe!

8. Cold Sheet
Your healing partner, if not 2 others, will need to help you out of the bathtub and right away begin wrapping you in the cold sheet that has been soaking in the bucket of ice. This will actually feel good. Don't wrap the sheet too tight. You don't want to feel claustrophobic.

Wear slippers from the bathroom to the bed to keep from losing any heat.

Lie down on your pre-prepared bed of plastic and 100% cotton sheets. Your healing partner will then cover you with another 100% cotton sheet followed by several non-synthetic blankets.

The cotton sheets will draw out old poisons that have come to your skin's surface as a result of the hot bath.

If you need to pee during the night, just pee in the sheet. It is not worth unwrapping and re-wrapping the sheets and blankets.

Stay wrapped up at least 3 hours, if not until morning. Someone will need to stay with you just in case you need anything, so you will not have to get up. By morning, the sheet may have turned multi-colored from all the poisons that have been drawn out through the skin. These toxins have been inside you for years – sometimes your whole life.

Keep your Cayenne Tincture and Lobelia Tincture close by in case you feel faint or have any cramps or spasms.

Note to your Healing Partner on the Emotional Release:
During that final 5 minutes in the tub, a lot of things can happen. I've seen people try and faint, but a dropper full of Cayenne Tincture in their mouth will ensure they're not going to lose consciousness. There is no way a person can faint with a mouth full of Cayenne Tincture. It's impossible. I've seen people go into whole body spasms and tetany. Lobelia Tincture ensures that you can stop them immediately without any lasting effects.

I've heard all the crying, screaming and fighting. It's a blessing that I spent 22 years in the martial arts, because with a few patients I needed all my abilities to keep them in the tub. Assure them that they're doing fine. Be strong, even stern if necessary. Keep them breathing, but keep them in the tub. This last five minutes may be the most important five minutes of the therapy. Something happens, I don't know exactly what, but a person may relive past trauma. The person may vomit. They may hallucinate. Don't be alarmed by this. Everything that happens at this point is perfect. Even if that means that green worms crawl out of their ears. Everything at this point is perfect and necessary for their healing. So trust and believe and keep a sense of humor about the whole thing.

I could give you one case about the emotional changes, but I'd have to give you a hundred. We all know that there's no such thing as just a physical disease. All diseases have their emotional rooting and emotional implications as well. I had hundreds of patients that had an emotional healing in that last five minutes of the treatment that was literally equal to a hundred years of psychotherapy and psychiatry. To say that these people were new individuals when they came out of the Cold Sheet Treatment would be an understatement. I don't tell you these stories to scare you or frighten you. No matter how intensely I cranked up the volume, I never saw anybody hurt or maimed by doing this treatment. What I did see were hundreds of people having miraculous healings.

Some people may consider this routine to be radical, but I assure you that it is not. Compared to anything that is done in a hospital, this routine is lightweight. All across America, people are suffering and dying at the hands of alternative healers and natural healers who don't have the guts to go beyond essential oils and massage and a mild diet to help someone recover from a killer disease. In the meantime, if this person goes to the hospital, the doctors are going to cut their legs off or cut their tumors out or do brain surgery. Anything that a hospital would do to treat the same disease would be a thousand times more painful, more aggressive, more intensive, and more invasive than the Cold Sheet Treatment.

> **"Tomorrow is what you believe and do today."**
>
> **– Dr. Richard Schulze**

A Few Case Histories on The Cold Sheet Treatment

When I first met Dr. Christopher, he had talked for years about hot and cold sheet treatments, but I had never seen it done. Shortly after meeting him, in the early days of my apprenticeship with him, I asked Dr. Christopher if I could please demonstrate it on a student. I had no idea what a powerful life-transforming treatment this would be for me as well as the student. After doing thirty or forty of these treatments on students each semester, I realized that I could make certain modifications to the program to make it both more intensive and easier to do. Dr. Christopher's instructions on the treatment had not come close to preparing me for what I would actually experience in giving this treatment to people.

Thyroid Cancer

I had a man with thyroid cancer come to a clinic that I was working at in England. He had a rapidly growing malignant tumor that totally wrapped around his thyroid. The doctors wanted to operate. They said that they would be removing his thyroid and would also be removing his larynx, and he would never speak again. In fact, the tumor was so large, that they wanted to remove a good portion of his entire throat. He asked if he could have a month to think about it, and they said that he could be dead within days. He decided not to undergo the surgery, and he came to the clinic. One of the first things we did with this man was give him the Cold Sheet Treatment. The tumor in his neck was approximately two inches wide when we measured it. The morning after his first Cold Sheet Treatment, the tumor had shrunk fifty percent to only one inch.

By the end of the week, the tumor was completely gone. It was obvious to me that the greatest impact at reversing this malignant cancer was the Cold Sheet Treatment. In fact, during the cold sheet, his last five minutes when he was screaming, I decided to do some deep body work on his throat from the outside and from the inside. At one point he vomited up a piece of this tumor. This was a tremendous healing for this man - certainly bypassing a lethal surgery that could have killed him. They would have removed his thyroid and destroyed his metabolism for the rest of his life, he would have had no energy and he would not have been able to speak because they would have removed his larynx.

He was so thrilled that he came back to the school for the next two years and paid his tuition just to sit in the classroom and tell the other students about his miraculous healing.

Lou Gehrig's Disease

I had a young woman who was diagnosed with A. Lateral Sclerosis, Lou Gehrig's disease, and possibly another nervous system degeneration like Parkinson's disease. She had tremors, muscle weakness and she was rapidly degenerating. I did a Cold Sheet Treatment on her and in the last five minutes, she went into the greatest full body spasm that I had ever seen. I believe that every muscle in her body went into a spasm at the same time. She turned into a hunk of iron. Now, you can imagine that this was extremely painful for her, but the Lobelia Tincture eased the spasms and the pain immediately. The next morning, this woman showed very few signs of having any neurologic disorders and by the end of the week she showed no signs at all. As far as I could see, she was completely healed. About two months later the doctors gave her a completely clean bill of health, to both the doctors' and her amazement.

rostate Cancer, Candida, Migraines, High Cholesterol, Endometriosis, Allergies, Poor
Disease, Memory loss, Blood Clots, Chronic Infections, Irritable Bowel Syndrome, Ch
Menopause, Herpes Simplex I II, Autoimmune Disorders, Anemia, Eczema, Epstein B
smitted Diseases, Alcoholism, Tremors, Benign Cysts and Tumors, Drug Addiction,
Depression, Fibrocystic Breast Disease, Chronic Diarrhea, Dermatitis, Hyperthyroid
Fibroids, Parasites, Pelvic Inflammatory Disease, Panic Attacks, Psoriasis, Lipomas
Candida, Skin Cancer, Rheumatoid Arthritis, Congestive Heart Failure, Kidney Fai
Strokes, Panic Attacks, Hypothyroidism, Lupus, HIV, Kidney Stones, Leukemia, CI
evere Burns, Gonorrhea, Schizophrenia, Seizures, Tuberculosis, Lead Poisoning, Pol
Disease, Multiple Sclerosis, Pyelonephritis, Pancreatic Cancer, Ulcerative Colit
tion, Brain Cancer, Juvenile Diabetes, Mitral Valve Prolapse, Syphilis, Crohn's Dise
Addison's Disease, Cirrhosis of the Liver, Scleroderma, Ovarian Cancer, Chlamydia,
ema, Lymphoma, Lou Gehrig's Disease, Gulf War Syndrome, Glaucoma, Liver Can
Myasthenia Gravis, Trichomonas, Nephrotic Syndrome, Rectal Cancer, Malaria, B
us Sclerosis, Polycystic Kidneys, Muscular Dystrophy, Lyme Disease, Sarcoidosis, Ray
Pituitary Tumors, Galactorrhea, Cystic Fibrosis, Colon Cancer, Parkinson's Disease,
ic Fatigue Syndrome, Breast Cancer, Depression, High Blood Pressure, Arthritis, Alzhe
, Asthma, Hepatitis, Cervical Cancer, Coronary Artery Disease, Migraines, Candia
esterol Endometriosis, Allergies, Poor Circulation, Heart Disease, Memory Loss, Blo
ic Infections, Irritable Bowel Syndrome, Chronic Sinusitis, Menopause, Herpes Simple
mmune Disorders, Anemia, Eczema, Epstein Barr, Sexually Transmitted Diseases, A
gn Cysts, Tumors, Drug Addiction, Infertility, Manic Depression, Fibrocystic Breas
ic Diarrhea, Dermatitis, Hyperthyroidism, Epilepsy, Uterine Fibroids, Parasites, Pel
Disease, Panic Attacks, Psoriasis, Lipomas, Food Allergies, Candida, Skin Cancer, I
ritis, Congestive Heart Failure, Kidney Failure, Lung Cancer, Strokes, Panic Attack
ism, Prostate Cancer, Lupus, HIV, Kidney Stones, Leukemia, Chronic Bronchitis, S
hea, Schizophrenia, Seizures, Tuberculosis, AIDS, Lead Poisoning, Polycystic Ovari
ultiple Sclerosis, Pyelonephritis, Pancreatic Cancer, Ulcerative Colitis, Atrial Fibri
rain Cancer, Juvenile Diabetes, Mitral Valve Prolapse, Syphilis, Crohn's Disease, C
ddison's Disease, Cirrhosis of the Liver, Emphysema, Scleroderma, Ovarian Cancer,
ar Degeneration, Retinitis Pigmentosa, Lymphoma, Lou Gehrig's Disease, Gulf War
oma, Liver Cancer, Stomach Cancer, Myasthenia Gravis, Trichomonas, Nephrotic S
l Cancer, Spinal Cord Injury, Malaria, Birth Defects, Tuberous Sclerosis, Polycystic
lar Dystrophy, Lyme Disease, Sarcoidosis, Raynaud's Disease, Pituitary Tumors, Ga
ibrosis, Colon Cancer, Parkinson's Disease, Diabetes, Chronic Fatigue Syndrome, Br
ssion, High Blood Pressure, Arthritis, Alzheimer's Disease, Asthma, Hepatitis, Cervic
onary Artery Disease, Migraines, Candida, High Cholesterol Endometriosis, Allergi
ation, Heart Disease, Memory Loss, Blood Clots, Chronic Infections, Irritable Bowel
nic Sinusitis, Menopause, Herpes Simplex I and II, Autoimmune Disorders, Anemia,
n Barr, Sexually Transmitted Diseases, Alcoholism, Tremors, Benign Cysts and Tum
on, Infertility, Cataracts, Macular Degeneration, Manic Depression, Fibrocystic Bre
c Diarrhea, Dermatitis, Hyperthyroidism, Epilepsy, Uterine Fibroids, Parasites, Pel
Disease, Panic Attacks, Psoriasis, Lipomas, Food Allergies, Candida, Skin Cancer, R
ritis, Congestive Heart Failure, Kidney Failure, Lung Cancer, Strokes, Fibromyalgi
ism, Prostate Cancer, Lupus, HIV, Kidney Stones, Leukemia, Chronic Bronchitis, S
hea, Schizophrenia, Seizures, Tuberculosis, AIDS, Lead Poisoning, Polycystic Ovari

CHAPTER 7

THE CIRCULATION
AND MOVEMENT PROGRAM

A. Massage/Bodywork

Massage the entire body every day with special emphasis on deep foot reflexology and all around the problem areas. Don't be afraid to touch your sore or sick parts. Put some life back into them.

Deep, painful, intense bodywork is O.K.

Crying and screaming is O.K.

All of this is better than the surgeon's knife.

B. Skin Brush

With a dry, natural plant-fiber skin brush, start at your feet and move upward toward your heart. Pay special attention to your affected areas as well as your lymph system in your groin area and under your arms. Don't forget your scalp and face. (Careful with the face.) SCRUB yourself thoroughly every day. Skin brushing stimulates the lymphatic flow. Your lymphatic system is the clear fluid of your body. It's the white blood and it contains pure immune cells. It doesn't have a pump like the heart, so skin brushing is one of the best ways to move that lymph around the body.

C. Exercise

You must exercise everyday. Do whatever you can, but push yourself to move. Increase the amount every day. You must breathe hard and work up a sweat. One hour each day is to be your eventual goal. If you rest, YOU RUST – EVEN ROT!

I don't care if you are paralyzed. I had a patient that was so paralyzed that they couldn't move anything except two fingers on each hand. So fine, I had them move and stretch those fingers, with deep breathing, 100 times, 3 times a day. The very next day they could move 4 fingers, and in no time the entire hand and arm. YOU HAVE TO START SOMEWHERE. I had another patient that could hardly move at all, so I had them just deep breathe and imagine moving. In a few days they were physically moving.

Don't let your excuses get in the way. MOVE!

D. Breathing

3-4 times a day do some deep breathing for at least 10 minutes. Deep breathing oxygenates your blood and stimulates your lymphatic and circulation systems.

...heimer's Disease, Asthma, Hepatitis, AIDS, Breast Cancer, Coronary
...state Cancer, Candida, Migraines, High Cholesterol, Endometriosis, Allergies, Poor C
...isease, Memory loss, Blood Clots, Chronic Infections, Irritable Bowel Syndrome, Chr
...Menopause, Herpes Simplex I II, Autoimmune Disorders, Anemia, Eczema, Epstein Ba
...mitted Diseases, Alcoholism, Tremors, Benign Cysts and Tumors, Drug Addiction, I...
...epression, Fibrocystic Breast Disease, Chronic Diarrhea, Dermatitis, Hyperthyroidis
...Fibroids, Parasites, Pelvic Inflammatory Disease, Panic Attacks, Psoriasis, Lipomas,
...andida, Skin Cancer, Rheumatoid Arthritis, Congestive Heart Failure, Kidney Fail
...Strokes, Panic Attacks, Hypothyroidism, Lupus, HIV, Kidney Stones, Leukemia, Ch
...vere Burns, Gonorrhea, Schizophrenia, Seizures, Tuberculosis, Lead Poisoning, Poly
...Disease, Multiple Sclerosis, Pyelonephritis, Pancreatic Cancer, Ulcerative Colitis
...ion, Brain Cancer, Juvenile Diabetes, Mitral Valve Prolapse, Syphilis, Crohn's Disea
...ddison's Disease, Cirrhosis of the Liver, Scleroderma, Ovarian Cancer, Chlamydia,
...ma, Lymphoma, Lou Gehrig's Disease, Gulf War Syndrome, Glaucoma, Liver Canc
...Myasthenia Gravis, Trichomonas, Nephrotic Syndrome, Rectal Cancer, Malaria, Bi
...s Sclerosis, Polycystic Kidneys, Muscular Dystrophy, Lyme Disease, Sarcoidosis, Ray
...Pituitary Tumors, Galactorrhea, Cystic Fibrosis, Colon Cancer, Parkinson's Disease,
... Fatigue Syndrome, Breast Cancer, Depression, High Blood Pressure, Arthritis, Alzher
...Asthma, Hepatitis, Cervical Cancer, Coronary Artery Disease, Migraines, Candida
...esterol Endometriosis, Allergies, Poor Circulation, Heart Disease, Memory Loss, Bloc
... Infections, Irritable Bowel Syndrome, Chronic Sinusitis, Menopause, Herpes Simple
...mune Disorders, Anemia, Eczema, Epstein Barr, Sexually Transmitted Diseases, A
...n Cysts, Tumors, Drug Addiction, Infertility, Manic Depression, Fibrocystic Breast
... Diarrhea, Dermatitis, Hyperthyroidism, Epilepsy, Uterine Fibroids, Parasites, Pelv
...Disease, Panic Attacks, Psoriasis, Lipomas, Food Allergies, Candida, Skin Cancer, R
...itis, Congestive Heart Failure, Kidney Failure, Lung Cancer, Strokes, Panic Attacks
...sm, Prostate Cancer, Lupus, HIV, Kidney Stones, Leukemia, Chronic Bronchitis, Se
...hea, Schizophrenia, Seizures, Tuberculosis, AIDS, Lead Poisoning, Polycystic Ovaria
...ultiple Sclerosis, Pyelonephritis, Pancreatic Cancer, Ulcerative Colitis, Atrial Fibrill
...rain Cancer, Juvenile Diabetes, Mitral Valve Prolapse, Syphilis, Crohn's Disease, Ch
...ddison's Disease, Cirrhosis of the Liver, Emphysema, Scleroderma, Ovarian Cancer,
...r Degeneration, Retinitis Pigmentosa, Lymphoma, Lou Gehrig's Disease, Gulf War
...oma, Liver Cancer, Stomach Cancer, Myasthenia Gravis, Trichomonas, Nephrotic S
... Cancer, Spinal Cord Injury, Malaria, Birth Defects, Tuberous Sclerosis, Polycystic
...ar Dystrophy, Lyme Disease, Sarcoidosis, Raynaud's Disease, Pituitary Tumors, Gal
...ibrosis, Colon Cancer, Parkinson's Disease, Diabetes, Chronic Fatigue Syndrome, Bre
...sion, High Blood Pressure, Arthritis, Alzheimer's Disease, Asthma, Hepatitis, Cervica
...nary Artery Disease, Migraines, Candida, High Cholesterol Endometriosis, Allergie
...tion, Heart Disease, Memory Loss, Blood Clots, Chronic Infections, Irritable Bowel S
...ic Sinusitis, Menopause, Herpes Simplex 1 and II, Autoimmune Disorders, Anemia,
... Barr, Sexually Transmitted Diseases, Alcoholism, Tremors, Benign Cysts and Tum
...n, Infertility, Cataracts, Macular Degeneration, Manic Depression, Fibrocystic Bree
... Diarrhea, Dermatitis, Hyperthyroidism, Epilepsy, Uterine Fibroids, Parasites, Pelv
...Disease, Panic Attacks, Psoriasis, Lipomas, Food Allergies, Candida, Skin Cancer, R
...itis, Congestive Heart Failure, Kidney Failure, Lung Cancer, Strokes, Fibromyalgia
...m, Prostate Cancer, Lupus, HIV, Kidney Stones, Leukemia, Chronic Bronchitis, Se
...hea, Schizophrenia, Seizures, Tuberculosis, AIDS, Lead Poisoning, Polycystic Ovaria

CHAPTER 8

CASTOR OIL PACKS, POULTICES AND FEMALE SUPPOSITORIES

Castor oil packs and the drawing poultices are for breaking up, dissolving and drawing our poisons, congestion and tumors.

Castor Oil Pack

Use the castor oil pack if you cannot feel the cancer or disease through the skin. Otherwise, use the black poultice that follows. Every evening, do a castor oil pack over the affected area and leave it on all night long. You can do multiple castor oil packs over different parts of the body. They can be kept warm with a hot water bottle. Soak a minimum one square foot piece of flannel. Heat the castor oil pack before you put it on. It's better to cover more of the area of you body than less. If you use more, you are cleansing the nearby areas, which are probably infected or congested also.

Go to your local fabric store and get some cotton muslin that's used for making baby diapers. They have it in big bolts. You can buy a whole bunch of it. Cut it up as you want. It helps to seam the edges. If this isn't thick enough, you can buy heavier weight cotton and kind of sandwich it in-between two pieces of the muslin. Then you can soak it in castor oil and have a really nice, thick pack. Or you can sew multiple layers of this together, or even put cotton batting inside.

Get some good cotton batting or cotton felt. Put one layer of cotton batting and one layer of muslin on each side and stitch together around the edges. This will absorb a lot of castor oil.

Cover the pack with plastic to keep it from soaking into your blankets and sheets. Eventually, the pack may get stained with colors from drawing out toxins. Change it with a fresh pack. It is not necessary to refrigerate the castor oil pack during the day.

Black Super Draw Poultice

If you can feel the tumor(s) through the skin, use the Black Super Draw Poultice. You will want to change it frequently. A drawing poultice removes impurities and poisons from the body, and can be more effective if changed 1 to 3 times a day.

Put the following ingredients in a blender
- 1 heaping handful of fresh red clover blossoms (if not available, use dried)
- 1/2 a handful of fresh chaparral leaf (if not available, use dried)
- 1/4 cup of fresh, grated poke root or 1/3 cup of the dried powder
- 2 tablespoons of goldenseal root powder
- 2 tablespoons of activated willow charcoal
- 1 teaspoon tea tree oil
- 1 teaspoon of bloodroot tincture
- 1 cup Bentonite clay
- 1 cup slippery elm inner bark

To heal and disinfect:
- Add 2 to 4 cloves of garlic

Important! If you have a malignant tumor resting just below the skin or starting to break through the skin, you may want to do serious surgery by adding:
- 1 entire bulb of peeled garlic cloves (at least 12 large cloves)
- If you are bleeding, add 1 tablespoon of Cayenne Powder or 5-10 dropperfuls of Cayenne Tincture

On the side, make a quart of liquid
- 50% raw organic apple cider vinegar
- 50% distilled water

This formulae is not written in stone. Feel free to add other blood cleansing and drawing herbs like fresh plantain.

Put the ingredients in a blender. Add enough 50/50 solution of distilled water and raw apple cider vinegar to make a thick, dryish paste. Blend well and apply.

If you are going to leave the poultice on all night long, apply about 1/2 inch of poultice, rub in well. To adhere, cover with cotton gauze and tape and then cover with a cotton towel or a piece of plastic if necessary.

I have used this cancer poultice hundreds, actually thousands, of times on all types of cancers, above and below the surface, with great results.

Poultices of this type have been used on cancers for hundreds of years and have proven very effective. This poultice is a general-purpose poultice for all types of cancers. One can never know whether a subdermal lump, bump, boil, cyst, tumor or toxic accumulation will break out and purge itself through the skin or be reabsorbed back into the body and eliminated internally. Either way, using a poultice over the area promotes speedy removal. This poultice greatly increases the blood flow and lymphatic circulation to the affected area and this in turn will help break up and disperse the congestion.

If the affected area is small like a wart, tiny cancer or boil, just slice a medium-to-large garlic clove in half and tape the flat, wet side of the garlic right on the spot. Tape it on with adhesive tape or a few Band-Aids and change the garlic 2 to 3 times daily. This will usually burn off what you want in a few days. Remember, GARLIC WILL BURN when used this way. Garlic contains sulfuric acid and will burn right through the skin. This can be helpful when you want to burn off cancers, warts, boils, or anything, but make sure you are also taking it internally.

After drawing out the cancer, there may be a hole in your body where you will want to regrow tissue with a healing poultice. Poultices are great for just about any problem but are mostly used for wounds. Before using a poultice on a "hole" in the body or a deep wound, you want to clean and disinfect the area as well. My favorite way is by swabbing on my Anti-Infection

Tincture. This will sting. Breathe. You can also add anti-infection herbs to the poultice, (Goldenseal, or my favorite, Garlic, which does burn a bit, or Tea Tree Oil). Another general rule of thumb for a wound is that once the poultice is dried, it may look like the poultice is gone or has been absorbed into the body. This one is NOT a drawing poultice, so, don't clean the remaining poultice off unless you absolutely need to recheck the wound. Just add a new poultice over the old one and keep "feeding" the area.

Recipes for Healing Poultices

My favorite healing poultice is fresh cut, older Aloe Vera leaves with the gel filleted out and applied directly to the area. IT'S THE BEST.

Aloe Vera is also one of my favorite additions to an herbal poultice. It adds soothing and healing qualities that help your body repair itself 2 to 10 times faster than normal. NOTE: There are literally thousands of Aloe Vera preparations sold all over the world. There are lotions, potions, gels, and liquids. I have NEVER, EVER seen ANY of them work at all – or do anything – period! ALL the miracles I've witnessed have been with the fresh plant only. To use Aloe Vera, pick a fresh leaf. This is done by just slicing the leaf off near the base of the plant with a sharp paring knife. The oldest leaves are at the base. These are the strongest. Take the leaf into the house and place on a cutting board. Trim off the leaf edges and then filet off the top and bottom skin until you are left only with a slab of clear gel. Place a slab of gel, at least 1/4 inch thick and not more than 1/2 inch thick, directly over the wound and hold it in place with cotton gauze and tape if necessary.

Herbal Healing Poultice
- 4 parts powdered slippery elm bark
- 2 parts powdered plantain leaf
- 1 part powdered goldenseal root
- 1 part powdered comfrey root
- A dash of powdered cayenne pepper

This poultice can be sprinkled directly into a wet or bloody wound in order to regrow new tissue, or it can be mixed it with warm water and applied to the area. For a healing poultice, you will notice that after some time, some of the poultice will look like it disappeared. This is good. This means your body has assimilated the herbs to make new tissue. Remember, don't rinse the herbs out of the wound, just keep adding more on top of what's already there.

Generally, once a poultice has dried on a wound, I consider it a part of the body. Just like a scab, it will come off in its own time.

A good example of this happened many years ago when I was with a woman who cut the tip of her finger entirely off. The finger was bleeding profusely, so I dumped a handful of cayenne pepper on it. When the bleeding stopped, (in about 2 seconds,) I put her fingertip on top of the cayenne pepper and just stuck it to the rest of her finger.

I covered the whole area with an herbal poultice made of mainly comfrey leaf and root, garlic, slippery elm and a few other herbs. After adding more of the poultice in the next few hours, I finally wrapped gauze around the whole area. The next morning, we realized that the poultice had dried hard with the gauze and she now had a rock hard herbal cast on her finger. I said not to worry. In about 3 days it worked itself off and we found a beautifully healed finger. The fingertip was reconnected with the finger. There was only slight redness around the cut area, but we could see lots of cayenne pepper under the new skin between the fingertip and the finger. I assured her that the body would digest the cayenne pepper over a few weeks. A month later, there was not even a scar.

"Stop judging. Celebrate everything. Yes, even your disease. It is your blessing."

– Dr. Richard Schulze

FEMALE SUPPOSITORIES

For women who have problems with cervical cancer and other diseases of the ovaries, uterus, and vagina. I suggest alternating between two different kinds of natural suppositories. One is just a simple insertion of a garlic clove. The other is an herbal suppository you can make at home.

Usually what I have them do is garlic cloves for a week and then the herbal suppositories for about a week. Or they could do 6 days garlic cloves, a day off, and then 6 days of the herbal suppositories.

They could also do a garlic on Monday, a suppository on Tuesday, a garlic on Wednesday or however they feel they would like to do it. But, at least do 6 days of the garlic cloves and 6 days of the suppositories during the 30-Day Program.

THE 6-DAY GARLIC SUPPOSITORY ROUTINE:

The garlic is done in 3 stages. Stage 1, the 1st night, you simply insert the garlic. The 2nd night, you bruise it. The 3rd night and thereafter, you cut slices into the garlic. Each stage is more intense than the last.

Stage 1 (The 1st night): Take a large garlic clove, the size of your thumb, peel it and insert it into the vagina and pull it out in the morning. To remove it, you just stand up; it will drop down and you pull out the garlic clove. **Make sure to use a large thumb size clove of Garlic the tiny gloves are more difficult to get out.**

Stage 2 (The 2nd night): Peel a large garlic clove, press on it, and bruise it. You bruise the garlic to activate a compound called allicin. The allicin in garlic does not exist unless you activate it. In other words, there isn't any allicin in garlic to begin with. There are only dry fiber cells and liquid acid cells. When you cut or crush garlic, the acid pours on the fiber and allicin is the result of that chemical reaction. What works in the garlic really isn't there until we chew it, or slice it, or bruise it. That is why fresh garlic cloves don't have much smell. But when you chop it up - boom, you're creating chemistry in your kitchen. So, press that garlic clove and bruise it and then insert it.

After bruising it, 99% of women won't notice any feeling in their vagina from the garlic.

Stage 3 (The 3rd night): Bruise the garlic and make some actual lateral slices with a knife in the clove. Now you're creating more allicin. Some women when they insert this sliced garlic will feel a slight tingling for about 5 minutes, but nothing major. That's okay; it won't hurt you at all. If it's too extreme, you can pull it out and make less slices and less bruises. Put that in and leave it in all night. Take it out in the morning.

Follow Stage 3 for the next 3 nights.

Do this 6-Day Garlic Routine and no bacteria, no fungus, no virus will be alive in your vaginal area. It will reduce the inflammation, and for those with cancer, we know that garlic destroys tumors.

Formula for vaginal suppositories:
Generally, we use this formula for vaginal infections, but it can be used all the way up to cancer of the cervix, endometrial cancer or whatever. You can customize it to your needs. In other words, if you have cancer, add poke root to the suppository. If not, you can skip it.

Here is what you will need:
- 16 ounce jar Coconut oil
- 2 bottle of Tea tree oil
- 2 ounces Goldenseal root finely powdered
- 2 ounces Yellow dock root finely powdered

Optional:
- Poke root
- Cayenne pepper
- Garlic

In a bowl mix 2 heaping tablespoons of finely powdered yellow dock and 2 heaping tablespoons of finely powdered goldenseal. Finely is a key word, because if you have rough herbs in there, it may be abrasive.

Add 4-6 dropperfuls of tea tree oil. Tea tree oil is a multi-spectrum antibiotic, and anti-fungal. It's an Australian shrub in oil form that is available commercially.

Put the jar of coconut oil in a pot of warm water. Coconut oil at room temperature is solid, but when you warm it up, it becomes liquid. Add enough coconut oil to the powdered herbs to create a dry pie-dough consistency. If it's too wet, when you go to make suppositories, they will lose their shape and turn into pancakes.

The key is to make the pie dough have a dry consistency and if you make it too wet, which everybody invariably does, just add more goldenseal and yellow dock. And if it's too dry, add more coconut oil. Just keep playing with it back and forth until you get a dry pie dough consistency.

Form the dry, herbal pie dough into 12 large or 24 medium suppositories. Place on a glass plate and put them in the freezer.

If you have cancer you can use equal parts poke root powder, yellow dock powder and goldenseal powder. If you are using fresh poke root you have to be really careful. You grate it through a kitchen grater. The poke root will be wet after being grated and will have a lot of acid in it and will burn you. Dry the grated poke root in a dry area or a dehydrator. Most people will sell it in a powder form and the powder is the least active, but also the least acid or burning.

Now, if you want to add something that's a little more dramatic, you can even put a slight pinch of cayenne in there. This is a powerful herb for really stimulating the blood flow. Remember, if we don't get the blood there, we are not going to get the healing we want. I'm talking about a very, very slight pinch here. And if we want to, we can add just a drop or two of garlic oil.

THE 6-DAY VAGINAL BOLUS ROUTINE:

When you take the suppositories out of the freezer, they will be frozen. You must insert the suppository within 30 seconds because when you hold on to them, they will start melting, just from your body heat. Grease up your vaginal area first with a little olive oil and then put the suppository in. You want to make sure you grease up first or it is a pretty rough ride.

The best way to do it is to put that suppository in at night; leave it in all night long. You will need to wear a sanitary napkin. Anyone who has vaginal problems should not use tampons.

In the morning, you'll notice a bit of that bolus is coming out. That's fine; leave it in all day long, then in the evening you want to do a douche. There's a couple of douches that are great to clean you all out. One of my favorites is a pint of water with a couple of tablespoons of fresh-squeezed lemon or lime juice. You can also use a couple of tablespoons of raw organic apple cider vinegar. Paul Braggs is an excellent brand of vinegar.

In the evening, put another bolus in. Follow this routine for six consecutive days.

Arthritis, Alzheimer's Disease, Asthma, Hepatitis, AIDS, Breast Cancer, Coronary
state Cancer, Candida, Migraines, High Cholesterol, Endometriosis, Allergies, Poor C
isease, Memory loss, Blood Clots, Chronic Infections, Irritable Bowel Syndrome, Chr
Menopause, Herpes Simplex I II, Autoimmune Disorders, Anemia, Eczema, Epstein Ba
mitted Diseases, Alcoholism, Tremors, Benign Cysts and Tumors, Drug Addiction, I.
epression, Fibrocystic Breast Disease, Chronic Diarrhea, Dermatitis, Hyperthyroidis
Fibroids, Parasites, Pelvic Inflammatory Disease, Panic Attacks, Psoriasis, Lipomas,
andida, Skin Cancer, Rheumatoid Arthritis, Congestive Heart Failure, Kidney Fail
Strokes, Panic Attacks, Hypothyroidism, Lupus, HIV, Kidney Stones, Leukemia, Ch
vere Burns, Gonorrhea, Schizophrenia, Seizures, Tuberculosis, Lead Poisoning, Poly
Disease, Multiple Sclerosis, Pyelonephritis, Pancreatic Cancer, Ulcerative Coliti
ion, Brain Cancer, Juvenile Diabetes, Mitral Valve Prolapse, Syphilis, Crohn's Disea
Addison's Disease, Cirrhosis of the Liver, Scleroderma, Ovarian Cancer, Chlamydia,
ma, Lymphoma, Lou Gehrig's Disease, Gulf War Syndrome, Glaucoma, Liver Canc
Myasthenia Gravis, Trichomonas, Nephrotic Syndrome, Rectal Cancer, Malaria, Br
s Sclerosis, Polycystic Kidneys, Muscular Dystrophy, Lyme Disease, Sarcoidosis, Ray
Pituitary Tumors, Galactorrhea, Cystic Fibrosis, Colon Cancer, Parkinson's Disease,
Fatigue Syndrome, Breast Cancer, Depression, High Blood Pressure, Arthritis, Alzhe
Asthma, Hepatitis, Cervical Cancer, Coronary Artery Disease, Migraines, Candid
esterol Endometriosis, Allergies, Poor Circulation, Heart Disease, Memory Loss, Bloc
Infections, Irritable Bowel Syndrome, Chronic Sinusitis, Menopause, Herpes Simple
mune Disorders, Anemia, Eczema, Epstein Barr, Sexually Transmitted Diseases, A
n Cysts, Tumors, Drug Addiction, Infertility, Manic Depression, Fibrocystic Breast
Diarrhea, Dermatitis, Hyperthyroidism, Epilepsy, Uterine Fibroids, Parasites, Pel
Disease, Panic Attacks, Psoriasis, Lipomas, Food Allergies, Candida, Skin Cancer, I
itis, Congestive Heart Failure, Kidney Failure, Lung Cancer, Strokes, Panic Attack
sm, Prostate Cancer, Lupus, HIV, Kidney Stones, Leukemia, Chronic Bronchitis, Se
bea, Schizophrenia, Seizures, Tuberculosis, AIDS, Lead Poisoning, Polycystic Ovari
ultiple Sclerosis, Pyelonephritis, Pancreatic Cancer, Ulcerative Colitis, Atrial Fibrill
ain Cancer, Juvenile Diabetes, Mitral Valve Prolapse, Syphilis, Crohn's Disease, Ch
ddison's Disease, Cirrhosis of the Liver, Emphysema, Scleroderma, Ovarian Cancer,
r Degeneration, Retinitis Pigmentosa, Lymphoma, Lou Gehrig's Disease, Gulf War
ma, Liver Cancer, Stomach Cancer, Myasthenia Gravis, Trichomonas, Nephrotic S
Cancer, Spinal Cord Injury, Malaria, Birth Defects, Tuberous Sclerosis, Polycystic
ar Dystrophy, Lyme Disease, Sarcoidosis, Raynaud's Disease, Pituitary Tumors, Ga
ibrosis, Colon Cancer, Parkinson's Disease, Diabetes, Chronic Fatigue Syndrome, Bre
sion, High Blood Pressure, Arthritis, Alzheimer's Disease, Asthma, Hepatitis, Cervic
nary Artery Disease, Migraines, Candida, High Cholesterol Endometriosis, Allergie
ation, Heart Disease, Memory Loss, Blood Clots, Chronic Infections, Irritable Bowel
ic Sinusitis, Menopause, Herpes Simplex I and II, Autoimmune Disorders, Anemia,
a Barr, Sexually Transmitted Diseases, Alcoholism, Tremors, Benign Cysts and Tum
n, Infertility, Cataracts, Macular Degeneration, Manic Depression, Fibrocystic Bre
Diarrhea, Dermatitis, Hyperthyroidism, Epilepsy, Uterine Fibroids, Parasites, Pel
Disease, Panic Attacks, Psoriasis, Lipomas, Food Allergies, Candida, Skin Cancer, I
itis, Congestive Heart Failure, Kidney Failure, Lung Cancer, Strokes, Fibromyalgi
sm, Prostate Cancer, Lupus, HIV, Kidney Stones, Leukemia, Chronic Bronchitis, Se
bea, Schizophrenia, Seizures, Tuberculosis, AIDS, Lead Poisoning, Polycystic Ovari

CHAPTER 9

ADDITIONAL ROUTINES

1. Every day, strip naked and take a sun and air bath for 10-15 minutes.

2. Every day take a walk outside in your bare feet and shuffle them in the grass or dirt – even lie down on the earth. Reconnect with nature and this planet you live on. If you are really bold, hug a tree.

3. Do deep breathing while you are outside. Fresh air will help you heal faster.

4. Use only natural soaps, shampoos, toothpastes and detergents.

5. Never use any deodorants, colognes, etc... You may use pure herbal essential oils if you smell.

6. If the odor is a problem, use my Clinical Air Treatment to cleanse and purify the air.

7. Wear only natural fiber clothing, cotton, wool, and silk. No polyester, nylon or blends.

HELPFUL HEALING TIPS

1. Read all this material top to bottom. Take a deep breath, then read it again!

2. Have all the supplies you will need for the entire 30-Day Program.

3. You must have a good support system. A friend to encourage you along the way, one that won't give into your "victim" stuff, your "why me" bull, somebody that will kick your butt when you need it. Another part of your support system will be my audios, videos, and anything I've written on natural healing. Embrace yourself. Surround yourself with natural healing. Read and re-read, watch and re-watch. You have to EAT, DRINK, SLEEP and BREATHE natural healing.

4. BEGIN and end each day by saying, "It's great to be alive, I love myself and I love my life."

5. HELP someone every day.

6. THROW OUT and give away 1/3 of everything you own. Bury your possessions before they bury you.

7. PRAY and MEDITATE.

8. Learn 1,000 jokes and LAUGH.

9. STOP watching ALL television, especially the news.

COMMONLY ASKED QUESTIONS

Q: Is this Program 30 days? A month? or 4 weeks long?

A: How about 4.3 weeks or 744 hours. Keep asking questions like that and you will never get well. Lighten up. Learn 1,000 jokes, or was it 1001?

Q: How long will it take me to get well?

A: Who knows? Try calling a psychic. Weather forecasters and stockbrokers make a living out of telling you the future. I don't. I have a question for you. How long did it take you to make yourself sick? How long have you been growing that tumor? Most of my patients got life changing results in 30 days. A few had to go 60 days and some 90 days or more. I have never heard ANY regrets.

Q: When I finish 30 days on the program, and I am not completely well, can I take a break or do I have to go right into the next 30 days?

A: A break of a few days or a week at most? Yes. A party? NO. Sure, depending on the severity of your disease, give yourself a break if you want to. You can relax a little. Sometimes a good break and a good rest is just as important to your healing as the program. Do not use this as an excuse to do anything that is harmful to you.

Q: Do I have to worry about mixing the different herbal formulae?

A: Many people are overly concerned about mixing the different herbal formulae. This is not necessary. Although you can hinder the effectiveness of the herbs, like using the female and male in the same mouthful, you can't hurt yourself. None of my patients ever blew themselves up. No explosions will occur. I tried to get all of my patients to look at herbal formulae in the same way they look at food. You never worry about eating a squash with a carrot thinking it might kill you. Herbs ARE foods and foods ARE herbs. It is true that herbs tend to have more concentrated amounts of plant chemicals in them, but they are still very safe to mix. Even industrial strength herbal formulae will tell you by their taste how much is enough. If you do overdose or mix badly, the worst outcome is usually nausea. If you are taking numerous different herbal formulae, like in this 30-Day Program, follow our daily chart and try to space them out as far as possible (a 1/2 hour is enough) and do not take too many in the same mouthful.

Q: Are there any problems consuming the alcohol in tinctures?

A: Occasionally a few people have an emotional or spiritual aversion to consuming alcohol. On this, I will make the following statements. The base of the majority of my tonics is mostly distilled water but they do have a pure organically grown grain alcohol or apple cider vinegar content. Grain alcohol dissolves and extracts certain important phytochemicals, plant chemicals that are necessary for the different formulae to be effective. Therefore, it is better than just water alone. For example, the diosgenin in Dioscorea Villousa (wild yam) is only soluble in alcohol and not in water. The alcohol also helps the herbs assimilate quickly into your body and preserves the formula which gives it an almost indefinite shelf life (over 5 years, if not over 50 years.)

The amount of alcohol per dose is insignificant. There is more in some mouthwashes. The amount of alcohol in the average dose of a tincture is equal to the amount of alcohol in a ripe banana. This dosage has been tested on people who are alcohol sensitive with no adverse reactions. I had many patients that were alcoholics on 12-step programs or in Alcoholics Anonymous that use tinctures without turning back into monsters again.

If you're still concerned about the alcohol, you can place the tincture in a cup, pour boiling water into it, and the alcohol will evaporate in seconds.

Q: I'm hypoglycemic or diabetic. Can I still juice fast? I've been told not to by my naturopath, doctor, etc...

A: Yes, this 30-Day Program has helped hundreds of diabetics cure their diabetes and get off insulin forever. Just be sensible and, as I mentioned in the Juice section, dilute your juices 50/50 with pure water.

Q: What do I do if my tumor bleeds when it's being drawn out by the poultice?

A: Add some Cayenne Powder to the poultice. You can even sprinkle a little cayenne powder right onto the open wound. Also remember to take the tincture internally.

Q: My doctor told me that I have an overactive immune system/auto-immune disease. Should I take echinacea, knowing that it stimulates the immune system?

A: Yes, you can take Echinacea. ALL of my patients took echinacea, and ALL of them got healed by using it. It's helpful to think of herbs more as balancers. Echinacea balances the immune system, helping it to work better at cleaning up the mess that is causing your disease in the first place.

Q: I'm afraid of stimulating my immune system too much. I've have heard that taking too much Echinacea will ruin my immune system.

A: I have never had anyone burn out their immune system using Echinacea. Echinacea is a powerful herb and you do need to take periodic breaks. This is why you take it for one week, then stop for one week during this 30-Day Program. It is similar to a round of antibiotics that you take for 7 day and then stop. I never had one patient with Echinacea poisoning or immune system burnout.

Q: If I'm very ill, do I have to wait and do your 3 month Foundational Program, first before doing the 30-day cleanse?

A: If you are seriously ill – maybe your doctor has told you that you only have weeks to months to live, I highly suggest you begin doing the 30-Day Intensive Cleansing and Detoxification Program immediately. Would you pour a cup of water on a raging fire, or would you use a fire hose? The 30-Day Program is the fire hose. Get to work.

> **"The first step in natural healing is RESPONSIBILITY. Natural Healing is about taking control of your life and being responsible for everything that goes in and out of your body, mind and spirit."**
> **– Dr. Richard Schulze**

DAILY SCHEDULE

This schedule is a suggested guideline. You can modify it to meet your personal needs. High enemas and the Cold Sheet Treatment are not on this daily schedule. You will need to add them to your weekly schedule. Also everyone needs to read Chapter 5, **"The Intestinal Detoxification Program,"** and add it to your daily schedule.

<u>**The night before:**</u> Soak 3-6 tablespoons of **Detoxification Herb Tea** OR 3 tablespoons of **Kidney/Bladder & Dissolve Tea Formula** in 60 ounces of distilled water as per directions on package.

7am
- Say a positive affirmation. Good Morning! It's great to be alive! I love my life!
- Drink 8 ounces distilled water.
- Start with **skin brushing,** then do the **Hot and Cold Shower Routine** with emphasis on the part of your body that is sick or hurting ending with cold.
- If you're using the **Super Black Draw Poultice,** rinse off yesterday's poultice in the shower and reapply a fresh one.

7:30
- Simmer **Detoxification Herb Tea** for 15 minutes per directions or simmer **Kidney/Bladder & Dissolve Tea Formula** for 1 minute.
- As tea is simmering, begin preparing **Liver Flush** in blender or the **Kidney Flush** per directions. You will be doing EITHER the Liver Flush or the Kidney Flush, not both.
- Drink Liver Flush or Kidney Flush; sit quietly to avoid any nausea. Strain tea and pour into mugs.

8:00
- 15 minutes after the Flush, drink the 2 cups of **Detoxification Herb Tea,** adding 2 dropperfuls of **Liver/Gall Bladder & Anti-Parasite Tonic Formula (L/G-AP)** or, if doing The Kidney Flush, drink 2 cups of **Kidney/Bladder & Dissolve Tea,** adding 2 dropperfuls of **Kidney/Bladder Formula.**

8:45	• Take **Intestinal Formula #2.** (1 heaping teaspoon in 8 ounces distilled water or juice followed by 8 ounces distilled water.)
9:15	• Take **D-TOX Formula** or **Echinacea Plus** (2 dropperfuls).
9:40	• Drink some diluted fruit or vegetable **juice** with **SuperFood.** • Take **Dr. Schulze's Cayenne Tincture or Powder.** Start with 5-10 drops 3 times per day or 1/8-1 teaspoon of the powder 3 times per day.
9:50	• Get some fresh air. Walk outside in bare feet. Get some **exercise,** and take some **deep breaths.**
11:00	• Drink more **juice** and/or potassium broth.
11:30	• Take **Intestinal Formula #2.** (1 heaping teaspoon in 8 ounces distilled water or juice followed by 8 ounces distilled water.)
12pm	• Eat lunch consisting of **raw juice or raw salad.** Take more Superfood with juice or sprinkle the dose on your salad. • Take at least 1 clove of garlic now and 2 more cloves later in the day.
1:00	• Drink 2 cups of **Detoxification Herb Tea,** adding 2 dropperfuls of **Liver/Gall Bladder & Anti-Parasite Tonic Formula (L/G-AP)** or, if doing The Kidney Flush, drink 2 cups of **Kidney/Bladder & Dissolve Tea,** adding 2 dropperfuls of **Kidney/Bladder Formula.** • Drink more **juice.** • Take some more of **Dr. Schulze's Cayenne Powder or Tincture** or juice a fresh, hot pepper with your juice. • **Massage** the sick part of your body at least once today or have someone do it for you.
1:20	• Repeat **D-TOX Formula** or **Echinacea Plus** (2 dropperfuls).

1:40	• Drink more juice and/or potassium broth.
2:15	• Take **Intestinal Formula #2.** (1 heaping teaspoon in 8 ounces water or juice followed by 8 ounces water.) • If using **Super Black Draw Poultice,** change and reapply it. • **Laugh** and tell some jokes!
2:45	• You guessed it! Drink more **juice.** • Forgive someone, or forgive yourself.
3:30	• Have at least 8-16 ounces of carrot juice some time today.
4:30	• Drink more **juice!** • Take more of **Dr. Schulze's Cayenne Tincture.** Build up dose gradually as tolerated.
4:45	• Drink 2 cups of **Detoxification Herb Tea,** adding 2 dropperfuls of **Liver/Gall Bladder & Anti-Parasite Tonic Formula (L/G-AP)** or, if doing The Kidney Flush, drink 2 cups of **Kidney/Bladder & Dissolve Tea,** adding 2 dropperfuls of **Kidney/Bladder Formula.** • Visualize the herbs going exactly to where they need to go to heal you.
5:00	• Repeat **D-TOX Formula** or **Echinacea Plus** (2 dropperfuls). • Take some more deep breaths. Imagine yourself well and what that feels like.
5:30	• Take **Intestinal Formula #2** (1 heaping teaspoon in 8 ounces distilled water or juice followed by 8 ounces distilled water.)
6:00	• Consume more juice or salad for dinner.
7:00	• Drink more **juice** (yes, again) or potassium broth.

8:00	• Do **The Hot and Cold Shower Routine** again ending with hot.
	• Drink <u>more</u> juice.
8:30	• Take **Intestinal Formula #2** (1 heaping teaspoon in 8 ounces distilled water or juice followed by 8 ounces distilled water.)
9:00	• Take **Intestinal Corrective Formula #1** with juice or food.
9:15	• Take **D-TOX Formula or Echinacea Plus** (2 dropperfuls).
9:45	• Begin soaking **Detoxification Herb Tea** for tomorrow. Take 2 dropperfuls of **Nerve Formula (N Formula)** if needed for sleep.
	• Apply **Castor Oil Pack** (or change and reapply **Super Black Draw Poultice**) to the part of your body that is sick or hurting.
	• Send your body some **healing messages** like, "I love being alive. My body is healing itself."
10:00	• Good night.
	• Imagine yourself well.
	• Job well done!

, Arthritis, Alzheimer's Disease, Asthma, Hepatitis, AIDS, Breast Cancer, Coronal
ostate Cancer, Candida, Migraines, High Cholesterol, Endometriosis, Allergies, Poor
Disease, Memory loss, Blood Clots, Chronic Infections, Irritable Bowel Syndrome, Ch
Menopause, Herpes Simplex I II, Autoimmune Disorders, Anemia, Eczema, Epstein E
smitted Diseases, Alcoholism, Tremors, Benign Cysts and Tumors, Drug Addiction,
Depression, Fibrocystic Breast Disease, Chronic Diarrhea, Dermatitis, Hyperthyroid
Fibroids, Parasites, Pelvic Inflammatory Disease, Panic Attacks, Psoriasis, Lipomas
Candida, Skin Cancer, Rheumatoid Arthritis, Congestive Heart Failure, Kidney Fa
Strokes, Panic Attacks, Hypothyroidism, Lupus, HIV, Kidney Stones, Leukemia, Cl
evere Burns, Gonorrhea, Schizophrenia, Seizures, Tuberculosis, Lead Poisoning, Pol
Disease, Multiple Sclerosis, Pyelonephritis, Pancreatic Cancer, Ulcerative Colit
tion, Brain Cancer, Juvenile Diabetes, Mitral Valve Prolapse, Syphilis, Crohn's Dise
Addison's Disease, Cirrhosis of the Liver, Scleroderma, Ovarian Cancer, Chlamydia,
ema, Lymphoma, Lou Gehrig's Disease, Gulf War Syndrome, Glaucoma, Liver Can
Myasthenia Gravis, Trichomonas, Nephrotic Syndrome, Rectal Cancer, Malaria, B
us Sclerosis, Polycystic Kidneys, Muscular Dystrophy, Lyme Disease, Sarcoidosis, Ray
Pituitary Tumors, Galactorrhea, Cystic Fibrosis, Colon Cancer, Parkinson's Disease,
c Fatigue Syndrome, Breast Cancer, Depression, High Blood Pressure, Arthritis, Alzhe
, Asthma, Hepatitis, Cervical Cancer, Coronary Artery Disease, Migraines, Candia
esterol Endometriosis, Allergies, Poor Circulation, Heart Disease, Memory Loss, Blo
c Infections, Irritable Bowel Syndrome, Chronic Sinusitis, Menopause, Herpes Simple
nmune Disorders, Anemia, Eczema, Epstein Barr, Sexually Transmitted Diseases, A
gn Cysts, Tumors, Drug Addiction, Infertility, Manic Depression, Fibrocystic Breast
c Diarrhea, Dermatitis, Hyperthyroidism, Epilepsy, Uterine Fibroids, Parasites, Pel
Disease, Panic Attacks, Psoriasis, Lipomas, Food Allergies, Candida, Skin Cancer, I
ritis, Congestive Heart Failure, Kidney Failure, Lung Cancer, Strokes, Panic Attack
sm, Prostate Cancer, Lupus, HIV, Kidney Stones, Leukemia, Chronic Bronchitis, Se
hea, Schizophrenia, Seizures, Tuberculosis, AIDS, Lead Poisoning, Polycystic Ovari
ultiple Sclerosis, Pyelonephritis, Pancreatic Cancer, Ulcerative Colitis, Atrial Fibril
rain Cancer, Juvenile Diabetes, Mitral Valve Prolapse, Syphilis, Crohn's Disease, Ch
ddison's Disease, Cirrhosis of the Liver, Emphysema, Scleroderma, Ovarian Cancer,
ar Degeneration, Retinitis Pigmentosa, Lymphoma, Lou Gehrig's Disease, Gulf War
oma, Liver Cancer, Stomach Cancer, Myasthenia Gravis, Trichomonas, Nephrotic S
l Cancer, Spinal Cord Injury, Malaria, Birth Defects, Tuberous Sclerosis, Polycystic
ar Dystrophy, Lyme Disease, Sarcoidosis, Raynaud's Disease, Pituitary Tumors, Ga
ibrosis, Colon Cancer, Parkinson's Disease, Diabetes, Chronic Fatigue Syndrome, Bre
ssion, High Blood Pressure, Arthritis, Alzheimer's Disease, Asthma, Hepatitis, Cervic
onary Artery Disease, Migraines, Candida, High Cholesterol Endometriosis, Allergie
ation, Heart Disease, Memory Loss, Blood Clots, Chronic Infections, Irritable Bowel I
ic Sinusitis, Menopause, Herpes Simplex I and II, Autoimmune Disorders, Anemia,
n Barr, Sexually Transmitted Diseases, Alcoholism, Tremors, Benign Cysts and Tum
n, Infertility, Cataracts, Macular Degeneration, Manic Depression, Fibrocystic Bre
: Diarrhea, Dermatitis, Hyperthyroidism, Epilepsy, Uterine Fibroids, Parasites, Pela
Disease, Panic Attacks, Psoriasis, Lipomas, Food Allergies, Candida, Skin Cancer, R
ritis, Congestive Heart Failure, Kidney Failure, Lung Cancer, Strokes, Fibromyalgia
sm, Prostate Cancer, Lupus, HIV, Kidney Stones, Leukemia, Chronic Bronchitis, Se
hea, Schizophrenia, Seizures, Tuberculosis, AIDS, Lead Poisoning, Polycystic Ovari
Sclerosis, Pyelonephritis, Pancreatic Cancer, Ulcerative Colitis, Atrial Fibril

CHAPTER 10

A NATURAL DEATH

We all eventually experience a physical death. For all of us this beautiful time will come. By using natural healing, herbs and my program, we are not trying to cheat death. We are increasing the quality and prolonging the quantity of life.

Medical universities tell us that the human body should last 125 years. We are lucky today if we make it to half that. There have been many people who lived to be 150, and even a few over 200. Looking at this miraculous being that we have been blessed with, I know that the ages in the Old Testament of the Bible are correct. I know that we could live 300, 400, 500 years – maybe more. I don't know if you or I will achieve this in our lifetime, but what about in 20 or 30 generations of better living?

When we finally die after living a healthy, natural lifestyle, what I have seen is that we go with no pain, a big smile on our face and in a room with our loved ones. Considering the screaming hospital death dramas, my patients prefer a natural death.

BIRTH AND DEATH AT HOME

One of the reasons we don't really live and enjoy our lives to the fullest is because we have hidden ourselves from the miracle of birth and the miracle of death. We now hide in hospitals and pay vast sums of money to be born and die in them because we are so afraid of the experience.

Birth and death are as much a part of life as everything in between and may actually be the best parts. Most of my patients denied themselves the beautiful experience of watching their families and loved ones be born and die. Because they missed these events they have created in themselves a false sense of immortality. This false sense of physical immortality promotes people to live boring, dull, mundane, uneventful, worthless lives and to not value life itself.

If we would bring birth and death back into our homes where they belong, we would all appreciate the gift of life much more and recognize the fragility and shortness of it. We would live life to the fullest, not hold back, dare to celebrate more and love more because we would be more present to the fact that we do not live forever.

I know that if we will dare to bring our birthing and our dying back into our homes, we would have more respect and reverence for all life. We would be less inclined to kill animals, to kill each other, and be more inclined to celebrate and love every day, every moment.

By bringing birth and death back into our homes and experiencing it we will change the world.

> **"Life is not a dress rehearsal. This is it. RIGHT NOW. You can choose to live it to the fullest or sit on the sidelines and watch it go by."**
> **– Dr. Richard Schulze**

Final Hour Regrets

In the many years I spent interviewing patients, not only in America but all over the world, I had the wonderful opportunity to talk with many elderly people. I also had the illuminating experience of being with many people just a few days, even a few hours before their death. For a few, I was the last person they saw. I must share with you that most of these visits were filled with regrets. The reason I'm telling you this is so you don't make the same mistakes.

What I heard was like a condensed version of their life. People have a tendency near death to look back at their life and examine it. What I heard were the many regrets for not living life to its fullest.

I don't remember ever hearing any regrets for believing too much, trusting too much, laughing too much or loving too much. All the regrets were based on holding back, not going far enough, not giving enough, not loving enough, not taking the chance, not saying what they wanted to say, not taking the risk, not living life totally.

Let's not wait until it is too late. Let's not have a list of unfulfilled wishes and unlived dreams as the final hour approaches. Take the chance, take the leap, dare to make this life rich. Love and live life to its fullest potential.

> **"Everyone dies. Not everyone really lives!"**
> — **Dr. Richard Schulze**

A Poem from Dr. Schulze's Dead Patients.

We screwed up.
Don't make our same mistakes. Don't hold back. Don't be stingy.
We all waited until it was too late
Now sitting on our death beds, gasping our last breath.

We all agreed. We wasted our lives. We didn't really live.
We would do anything for a few more hours,
But all we can do is warn you,
Tell you that you are making the same mistakes we did.

We regret letting our fear and complacency rule us.
We didn't go far enough. We didn't live enough.
We didn't love enough. We didn't take enough chances.
We kept our mouths shut and didn't say what we really wanted to say.

We should have trusted more, believed more,
Laughed more, loved more.
We should have taken more risks, lived life to the fullest,
Traveled more, worked less and had more sex.

It's too late for us. We have so many unfulfilled wishes
And so many unlived dreams.
Please don't make our same mistakes.
Take the chance. Take the leap. Love Life and Live Life to the fullest

rostate Cancer, Candida, Migraines, High Cholesterol, Endometriosis, Allergies, Poor
Disease, Memory loss, Blood Clots, Chronic Infections, Irritable Bowel Syndrome, Cl
Menopause, Herpes Simplex I II, Autoimmune Disorders, Anemia, Eczema, Epstein
smitted Diseases, Alcoholism, Tremors, Benign Cysts and Tumors, Drug Addiction,
Depression, Fibrocystic Breast Disease, Chronic Diarrhea, Dermatitis, Hyperthyroid
Fibroids, Parasites, Pelvic Inflammatory Disease, Panic Attacks, Psoriasis, Lipoma
Candida, Skin Cancer, Rheumatoid Arthritis, Congestive Heart Failure, Kidney Fa
Strokes, Panic Attacks, Hypothyroidism, Lupus, HIV, Kidney Stones, Leukemia, C
evere Burns, Gonorrhea, Schizophrenia, Seizures, Tuberculosis, Lead Poisoning, Po
Disease, Multiple Sclerosis, Pyelonephritis, Pancreatic Cancer, Ulcerative Colit
tion, Brain Cancer, Juvenile Diabetes, Mitral Valve Prolapse, Syphilis, Crohn's Dis
Addison's Disease, Cirrhosis of the Liver, Scleroderma, Ovarian Cancer, Chlamydia
ema, Lymphoma, Lou Gehrig's Disease, Gulf War Syndrome, Glaucoma, Liver Ca
Myasthenia Gravis, Trichomonas, Nephrotic Syndrome, Rectal Cancer, Malaria, I
us Sclerosis, Polycystic Kidneys, Muscular Dystrophy, Lyme Disease, Sarcoidosis, Ra
Pituitary Tumors, Galactorrhea, Cystic Fibrosis, Colon Cancer, Parkinson's Disease
ic Fatigue Syndrome, Breast Cancer, Depression, High Blood Pressure, Arthritis, Alzh
e, Asthma, Hepatitis, Cervical Cancer, Coronary Artery Disease, Migraines, Candi
lesterol Endometriosis, Allergies, Poor Circulation, Heart Disease, Memory Loss, Bl
ic Infections, Irritable Bowel Syndrome, Chronic Sinusitis, Menopause, Herpes Simp
mmune Disorders, Anemia, Eczema, Epstein Barr, Sexually Transmitted Diseases,
gn Cysts, Tumors, Drug Addiction, Infertility, Manic Depression, Fibrocystic Breas
ic Diarrhea, Dermatitis, Hyperthyroidism, Epilepsy, Uterine Fibroids, Parasites, Pe
Disease, Panic Attacks, Psoriasis, Lipomas, Food Allergies, Candida, Skin Cancer,
ritis, Congestive Heart Failure, Kidney Failure, Lung Cancer, Strokes, Panic Attac
ism, Prostate Cancer, Lupus, HIV, Kidney Stones, Leukemia, Chronic Bronchitis, S
rhea, Schizophrenia, Seizures, Tuberculosis, AIDS, Lead Poisoning, Polycystic Ovar
Multiple Sclerosis, Pyelonephritis, Pancreatic Cancer, Ulcerative Colitis, Atrial Fibri
rain Cancer, Juvenile Diabetes, Mitral Valve Prolapse, Syphilis, Crohn's Disease, C
Addison's Disease, Cirrhosis of the Liver, Emphysema, Scleroderma, Ovarian Cance
ar Degeneration, Retinitis Pigmentosa, Lymphoma, Lou Gehrig's Disease, Gulf War
coma, Liver Cancer, Stomach Cancer, Myasthenia Gravis, Trichomonas, Nephrotic
al Cancer, Spinal Cord Injury, Malaria, Birth Defects, Tuberous Sclerosis, Polycysti
lar Dystrophy, Lyme Disease, Sarcoidosis, Raynaud's Disease, Pituitary Tumors, Ge
ibrosis, Colon Cancer, Parkinson's Disease, Diabetes, Chronic Fatigue Syndrome, B
ssion, High Blood Pressure, Arthritis, Alzheimer's Disease, Asthma, Hepatitis, Cervi
onary Artery Disease, Migraines, Candida, High Cholesterol Endometriosis, Allerg.
ation, Heart Disease, Memory Loss, Blood Clots, Chronic Infections, Irritable Bowel
nic Sinusitis, Menopause, Herpes Simplex I and II, Autoimmune Disorders, Anemia
n Barr, Sexually Transmitted Diseases, Alcoholism, Tremors, Benign Cysts and Tun
ou, Infertility, Cataracts, Macular Degeneration, Manic Depression, Fibrocystic Br
c Diarrhea, Dermatitis, Hyperthyroidism, Epilepsy, Uterine Fibroids, Parasites, Pe
Disease, Panic Attacks, Psoriasis, Lipomas, Food Allergies, Candida, Skin Cancer,
ritis, Congestive Heart Failure, Kidney Failure, Lung Cancer, Strokes, Fibromyalg
ism, Prostate Cancer, Lupus, HIV, Kidney Stones, Leukemia, Chronic Bronchitis, S
hea, Schizophrenia, Seizures, Tuberculosis, AIDS, Lead Poisoning, Polycystic Ovar

CHAPTER 12

A BIOGRAPHY OF
DR. RICHARD SCHULZE

Dr. Richard Schulze is one of the foremost authorities on natural healing and herbal medicines in the world. He operated a Natural Healing Clinic, first in New York, and later in Southern California for almost 20 years. For the past 17 years, he has continued to teach throughout the United States, Canada, Europe and Asia. He has designed natural therapy programs, which have assisted tens of thousands of people to create miracles and regain their health.

When he was 11 years old, Dr. Schulze's father died in his arms from a major heart attack. At 14, his mother also died of a heart attack. They were each only 55 years old. At age 16, Richard was diagnosed with an "incurable" genetic heart deformity. The doctors said he would be dead by the age of 20. After curing himself of this so-called "incurable" disease through changes in his lifestyle, and NO surgery, he set out on a mission to help others. He continues this healing mission today through his daily work to reveal the truth and the unlimited healing power of our being. He continues to teach on the use of herbs and the fundamentals of natural healing to help people to help themselves. He is also a leader in exposing fraud in medical, pharmaceutical and even herbal industries.

He is considered an innovator, a purist, even an extremist by many of his colleagues, but to his patients he is considered, "The man who has the guts to say and do what the others are afraid to." In the field of natural healing, he dared to pioneer new techniques and therapies which went far beyond what most people thought possible with alternative medicine. The outcome of his work has been the achievement of miraculous and unprecedented results. His herbal formulae and 30-Day Cleansing and

Detoxification Program are used at clinics worldwide to help people heal themselves from degenerative diseases such as Heart Disease, Cancer, Arthritis and A.I.D.S. The positive results have caused reverberations in both the natural and medical communities.

Dr. Schulze assisted and taught for the late Dr. John Christopher. After Dr. Christopher's death, Dr. Schulze continued to teach at his school for over 12 years. He has served as the Director of The College of Herbology and Natural Healing in the United Kingdom for 11 years and is also Co-Director of The Osho School for Naturopathic Medicine in France. Dr. Schulze has taught and lectured at numerous universities including Cambridge and Oxford Universities in England, Trinity Medical College in Ireland, Omega Institute in New York, Cortijo Romero in Spain and other natural therapy and herbal institutes worldwide. He has been the guest speaker on numerous radio and television shows in the United States and Europe. As a teacher he is loved for his intensity, passion, dedication to students, sense of humor, creativity, and his exciting, enthusiastic and evangelistic teaching style. He is mostly recognized for his unequaled understanding of natural healing.

Dr. Schulze is the creator of The American Botanical Pharmacy's line of industrial-strength, pharmaceutical, botanical extracts. He has manufac-tured these herbal products in the United States and in Europe for 20 years. His herbal formulae are famous for their strength and efficacy.

Dr. Schulze served an internship with the famous natural healer Dr. Bernard Jensen and apprenticed with the late Dr. John Christopher, grad-uating to teach side by side with Dr. Christopher for many years. Besides having a Doctorate in Herbology from The School of Natural Healing and a Doctorate in Natural Medicine he also holds a degree in Herbal Pharmacy and three degrees in Iridology. He is certified in eight different styles of Body Therapy and holds three black belts in the Martial Arts. He has written many clinical research papers on the topics of Botanical

Pharmacognosy, Pharmacology and the making of Herbal Preparations. He has written for Sam Biser's famous newsletter, has recorded many video and audio tapes and has co-authored books in Europe.

HERBAL SUPPLY LIST

AMERICAN BOTANICAL PHARMACY – *The exclusive manufacturer of Dr. Schulze's Original Clinical Formulae Organic and Wild Harvested Herbal Preparations*
    Mailing address: P.O. Box 9699
    Marina Del Rey, California 90292
    Retail Outlet: 4143 Glencoe Avenue
    Marina Del Rey, California 90292
    Telephone: 1-800-HERB-DOC

PACIFIC BOTANICALS *(Minimum 1 pound bulk herbs)*
    4350 Fish Hatchery Road
    Grants Pass, Oregon 97527
    Telephone: 1-541-479-7777

HORIZON HERBS *(Medicinal Herbal Seeds only)*
    P.O. Box 69
    Wilhams, Oregon 97544
    Telephone: 1-541-846-6704

NATURAL ❧ HEALING
PUBLICATIONS
BOOKS, AUDIOS AND VIDEOS

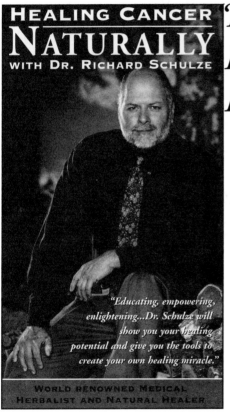

HEALING CANCER NATURALLY
WITH DR. RICHARD SCHULZE

"Educating, empowering, enlightening...Dr. Schulze will show you your healing potential and give you the tools to create your own healing miracle."

WORLD RENOWNED MEDICAL HERBALIST AND NATURAL HEALER

'Educating, Empowering and Enlightening..."

Dr. Schulze will show you your healing potential and give you the tools to create your own healing miracle.

This four tape audio series features Dr. Richard Schulze lecturing on *Healing Cancer Naturally* from Seattle, WA, where 450 people from 12 different states came to learn how he helped his patients heal their cancer, and not get it back. Others came to celebrate because they healed their cancer using Dr. Schulze's programs. **4 audio tapes:** $35.00

"There are **NO** incurable diseases. If you're willing to take responsibility for yourself and your life, you can heal yourself of anything."
— Dr. Richard Schulze

TO ORDER CALL TOLL FREE 1-877-TEACH-ME (1-877-832-2463)

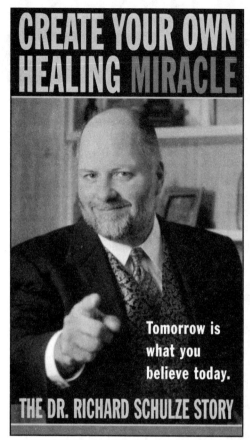

CREATE YOUR OWN HEALING MIRACLE

Tomorrow is what you believe today.

THE DR. RICHARD SCHULZE STORY

CREATE YOUR OWN HEALING MIRACLE
THE DR. RICHARD SCHULZE STORY

In this incredible 2 hour video Dr. Schulze tells how he healed himself of a killer heart disease, 4th degree burns and a crippling knee injury. The doctors said he would be dead by age 20 without open heart surgery, never grow his skin back without multiple skin graft operations and never walk again without extensive knee surgery. Watch how he proved them wrong.

This tape includes 45 minutes of live, unsolicited testimonials by people who were told that without surgery, drugs, chemotherapy or radiation they would be sick the rest of their lives. Some were even sent home to die. These people know the awesome healing power of Dr. Schulze's programs first hand, because, against all odds, they created their own HEALING MIRACLES. This video will inspire you to take control of your health and CREATE *YOUR OWN* PERSONAL HEALING MIRACLE

2 HOUR VIDEO: **$15.00**

IF YOU'RE TRYING TO CONVINCE SOME-ONE NATURAL HEALING WORKS...THIS VIDEO WILL DO IT!

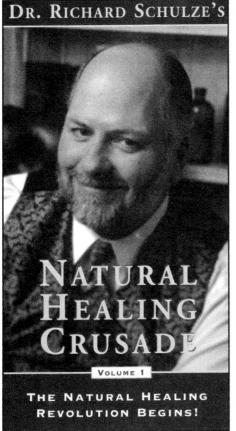

DR. RICHARD SCHULZE'S
NATURAL HEALING CRUSADE

Filmed live in California at one of Dr. Schulze's Natural Healing Crusades, these tapes are filled with Dr. Schulze's Natural Healing power, enthusiasm, wisdom, and passion. He describes ALL of his Foundational Natural Healing programs in detail. It's like having him right in your living room. In this video series, he will give you the same step-by-step instructions he gave to every one of his patients in his clinic.

In this 8 video series Dr. Schulze covers: ➤ The Fundamentals of Natural Healing ➤ Determining your level of health ➤ Creating Super Health and healing yourself from any disease ➤ The causes behind all disease and how to eliminate them ➤ The Elimination Organs and Intestinal Detoxification Program ➤ Dr. Schulze's 3 Healing Food Programs ➤ Juice Flushing ➤ Dr. Schulze's Movement, Circulation and Hydrotherapy Programs and ➤ Healing yourself using the power of your Mind and Emotions

8 VIDEOTAPE SERIES: $125.00

ORDER FORM

QTY.	BOOK	PRICE
	THERE ARE NO INCURABLE DISEASES - Dr. Schulze's 30-Day Intensive Cleansing and Detoxification Program **$12.00**	

QTY.	AUDIO TAPES	PRICE
	HEALING CANCER NATURALLY – 4 audio tape series *Includes FREE book! "There Are No Incurable Diseases"* **$35.00**	

QTY.	VIDEO TAPES	PRICE
	CREATE YOUR OWN HEALING MIRACLE The Dr. Richard Schulze Story – 2 hour video **$15.00**	
	DR. SCHULZE'S NATURAL HEALING CRUSADE 8 VIDEOTAPE SERIES **$125.00**	

SUBTOTAL		
Sales tax for CA residents in L.A. County . . . . 8.25% *Sales tax for CA residents outside L.A. County 7.25%*		
Orders between $1.00 and $99.99 add $5.00 postage	*$5.00*	
Orders between $100.00 and $199.99 add $6.50 postage	*$6.50*	
Orders between $200.00 and $299.99 add $8.50 postage	*$8.50*	
Orders over $300.00 add $10.00 postage	*$10.00*	
TOTAL DUE	**$**	

PLEASE PRINT CLEARLY AND USE BLOCK LETTERING

Name:

Ship to address:

City, State, Zip Code:

Daytime Phone: *Evening Phone:*

Name as it appears on your Credit Card:

Credit Card Number (MC, Visa, Amex, Discover):   *Exp. Date:*

☐ *I'm including a check or money order payable to Natural Healing Publications*

TO ORDER CALL TOLL-FREE 1-877-TEACH-ME (832-2463)